I Have Cancer:
What Should I Do?

Your Orthomolecular Guide for Cancer Management

Michael J. González, D.Sc., Ph.D.
Jorge R. Miranda-Massari, Pharm.D.
Andrew W. Saul, Ph.D.

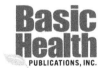
Basic Health
PUBLICATIONS, INC.

The information contained in this book is based upon the research and personal and professional experiences of the authors. It is not intended as a substitute for consulting with your physician or other healthcare provider. Any attempt to diagnose and treat an illness should be done under the direction of a healthcare professional.

The publisher does not advocate the use of any particular healthcare protocol but believes the information in this book should be available to the public. The publisher and authors are not responsible for any adverse effects or consequences resulting from the use of the suggestions, preparations, or procedures discussed in this book. Should the reader have any questions concerning the appropriateness of any procedures or preparation mentioned, the authors and the publisher strongly suggest consulting a professional healthcare advisor.

Basic Health Publications, Inc.
www.basichealthpub.com

Library of Congress Cataloging-in-Publication Data
Gonzalez, Michael J.
  I have cancer, what should I do? : your orthomolecular guide for cancer management / Michael J. Gonzalez, Jorge R. Miranda-Massari, Andrew W. Saul.
    p. cm.
  Includes bibliographical references and index.
  ISBN 978-1-59120-243-1 (Pbk.)
    1. Cancer—Diet therapy—Popular works. 2. Cancer—Chemotherapy—Popular works.
  3. Orthomolecular therapy—Popular works. I. Miranda-Massari, Jorge R. II. Saul, Andrew W. III. Title.
  RC271.V58G66 2009
  616.99'40654—dc22
                                          2009021243

Editor: John Anderson
Typesetting/Book design: Gary A. Rosenberg
Cover design: Mike Stromberg

ISBN 978-1-68162-737-3 (Hardcover)

Contents

*This book is dedicated to
the memory of Juan Guzmán,
Luz Leandry, Daisy Guzmán,
José R. Miranda, Miriam Alfaro,
Aida Massari, Laban Chamberlin,
and to our mentors,
Dr. Abram Hoffer, Dr. Harold D. Foster,
and Dr. Hugh D. Riordan.*

Acknowledgments

There are many people that we would like to thank—too many to mention—so here's a short list:

Inés Alfaro, M.D., kindly assisted us with case histories. She is a survivor of advanced breast cancer and that's how she learned about integrative medicine. Our thanks to Dr. Erik Paterson for his excellent and encouraging article. We also thank the late Abram Hoffer, M.D., Ph.D., for contributing the foreword to this book and providing over five decades of expert guidance and an example to all orthomolecular practitioners.

We also would like to express our gratitude to Dr. James A. Jackson for his pivotal role in the advancement of nontoxic cancer therapies, especially intravenous vitamin C, and for his ongoing collaboration and support.

Finally, we would like to thank our editor, John Anderson, for his professionalism, patience, and dedication to this book project.

Foreword

Very few diagnoses shock patients as much as being told that they have cancer. Cancer is a modern pandemic sweeping around the world. In developed countries, about half the total number of deaths are caused by cancer.

But when a few patients accept this diagnosis as a major challenge, they are often defeated by the attitude of their oncologist and leave the oncologist's office feeling depressed, disheartened, and defeated. I have seen over 1,500 cancer patients since 1976 and they've shared with me how they were treated. It is difficult to find a sympathetic doctor who knows how to deal with serious diseases and can encourage their patients to remain hopeful and thinking of recovery. Oncologists have seen few recoveries and their reaction is based on their professional experience of failure. Unfortunately, too few patients have heard that cancer is not necessarily always a killer disease and that in many cases it can be controlled with orthomolecular (nutritional) methods combined with orthodox treatment and with proper support from doctors, family, and friends.

Oncologists have to learn not to destroy hope. It is essential that patients not be deprived of hope even with what appears to be terminal cases. I have seen too many of these so-called hopeless cases recover. Like the middle-aged woman who had a severe kidney cancer that had spread into her back and surrounded her aorta. Surgery was impossible and she was entered into hospice care, with the usual grim prognosis. She came to see me and was started on the orthomolecular program described in this book. Two years later, a hospice nurse called to tell me that the patient was being discharged (the nurse considered this a miracle as she had never seen this happen before). Today, six years later, she is still well.

Based upon my experience with a large number of patients over the past thirty years—mostly terminal cases, many of whom were cured (no recurrence in ten years) or had their lives extended many years—I am convinced that every cancer patient deserves a chance for recovery, which orthomolecular treatment provides. Usually they feel better within a few days after they start taking vitamin C and they continue to feel better. Vitamin C is the major healing factor but many other nutrients, such as niacin, are also therapeutic.

One of the problems is the erroneous notion held by oncologists that antioxidants like vitamin C prevent the therapeutic action of chemotherapy and radiation. This is based entirely on bad hypotheses. Vitamin C is blamed even though every investigator who has studied this issue concluded that not only is it not toxic but it improves the treatment outcome and decreases the usual side effects of conventional treatments.

This book shows that ascorbic acid (vitamin C) used in optimum doses does not decrease the therapeutic effect of chemotherapy and radiation. There is so little clinical evidence that chemotherapy is actually efficacious for most cancers that it is difficult to conclude that ascorbic acid decreases the effect. Also, vitamin C protects the patient against some of the side effects of the treatment and increases the therapeutic response. Fortunately, a few oncologists have developed some insight and no longer have that conviction about the potential dangers of natural antioxidants like vitamins. This book will increase the number, if only they can be persuaded to read it.

—Abram Hoffer, M.D., Ph.D.

Preface

"Hell isn't merely paved with good intentions;
it's walled and roofed with them. Yes, and furnished too."
—ALDOUS HUXLEY (1894–1963)

This book is not intended as a substitute for appropriate medical care but as a complement to such care. Please keep the following in mind as you read:

- Do not self-diagnose. It is important to question and to be informed. It is important to get involved with your health care. Appropriate medical care is also critical for good health. If you have any concern about what is discussed in this book, please consult a health-care practitioner that you trust. Do not guess.

- Make your physician aware of all nutritional supplements or herbal products you are using to avoid undesirable interactions.

- Educate yourself. Use reliable sources of information and verify and re-evaluate. This is a field of rapid developments and not all licensed health-care practitioners are knowledgeable of the vast and complicated field of dietary supplements.

- If you are currently taking prescription medicine, please work with your doctor before making any change in your current treatment.

- Cancer is a multifactorial disease that requires a multifactorial treatment plan: medical, nutritional, and lifestyle changes as well as mental, emotional, social, and spiritual support. You cannot just take some pills and not change your diet, or change the diet and ignore important emotional or spiritual issues in your life, and then expect that everything will be fine. Any effective approach for cancer must be truly integrated. Otherwise, even if you get a response, you may still be setting the stage for cancer to come back.

This book is intended to give you valuable information on how to deal with cancer and improve your overall health. We will emphasize nutritional and orthomolecular strategies to improve your overall strength and to avoid the spread of cancer. We will also mention other important factors that need to be addressed in order to successfully manage cancer.

> *"The evil that is in the world almost always comes of ignorance,*
> *and good intentions may do as much harm as malevolence*
> *if they lack understanding."*
> —ALBERT CAMUS (1913–1960)

CHAPTER 1

Not a Death Sentence

*"It is impossible for anyone to begin to learn
what he thinks he already knows."*
—EPICTETUS (CA. 55–CA. 135)

For most people, the idea that they have cancer is truly frightening. The reason for this fright is that many people still die of cancer in spite of receiving the most advanced medical treatment in the most renowned medical centers. Often, those who are lucky survivors suffer the harsh physical, mental, and emotional consequences of the medical treatment of cancer. I (Jorge) recall the feeling of confusion we had when trying to decide on a course of action when a breast cancer diagnosis was confirmed for my wife. If medical education is uniform and the standard of care is so well-established, how can we have such a wide range of opinions, even among specialists?

What about all the people who shared information with me about how a family member or friend saved their lives by recommending a certain diet, vitamin, or a herbal remedy? How can so many people have so many different successful remedies? Are these myths? Could those remedies also cause harm?

We think it takes science to untangle the truth. One of the problems with the medical treatment of cancer (as with the treatment of many other conditions) is that the scientific knowledge is not well integrated, and it often takes too long to be accepted and applied. In the case of people with a potentially lethal disease, a wise balance between risk and benefit should always be made, but this is often not the case. There are many nutrition-based strategies that are well-established as

1

nontoxic and that can provide substantial benefits to the patient. Yet they are frequently ignored and even discouraged because of misinformation and ignorance, not only in the lay public but also among health professionals.

BE WELL INFORMED

In order for you to make responsible decisions, you need to be well informed and consider the implications of your decisions in terms of your own health and values. Despite what is written in the mission statement of the U.S. Food and Drug Administration (FDA) (www.fda.gov/AboutFDA/WhatWeDo/default.htm), this agency does not promote the approval of the most efficacious, least toxic, and most cost-effective treatments. The types of claims the FDA allows on labels differ between dietary supplements and drugs. The claims allowed for drugs have to do with diseases, while the claims allowed in the dietary supplements can only include the relation of the substance with the integrity of body's structures or normal function. If there is a dietary supplement that can maintain the integrity of cartilage and improve the function of the joints, you cannot say it helps in arthritis, even though it is obvious that it does.

Clinicians are not required to inform patients of alternative treatments, even if those treatments are more effective, less expensive, and have fewer side effects than conventional treatments. Medical practitioners do not use nutritional supplements because they were not taught about this in medical school, and it is not commonly presented in continuing education conferences or in the most commonly read medical journals. Medical practice is based on guidelines created by groups of prestigious specialists who rarely have a command of scientific and medical literature in the areas of nutritional supplementation, mind–body medicine, or psychoneuroendocrinology. This situation is difficult to change because it is driven by strong economic influences—particularly the powerful and profitable pharmaceutical industry—that flow to medical schools, medical associations, insurance companies, and through lobbying our government.

A basic principle of therapeutics, usually taught during the first few

Undue Influence of Drug Companies

"Is there some way (drug) companies can rig clinical trials to make their drugs look better than they are? Unfortunately, the answer is yes. Trials can be rigged in a dozen ways, and it happens all the time." This uncompromising statement comes from Dr. Marcia Angell, former editor-in-chief of the *New England Journal of Medicine,* in her book *The Truth About the Drug Companies* (New York: Random House, 2004). A highly respected and established medical insider, she does not shrink from attacking an industry which, she says, "will do almost anything to protect exclusive marketing rights."

Dr. Angell shows that clinical trials are often fixed. One way to load the dice, she writes, "is to enroll only young subjects in trials, even if the drugs being tested are meant to be used mainly in older people. Because young people generally experience fewer side effects, drugs will look safer." Another of the common ways to bias trials is to "present only part of the data—the part that makes the product look good—and ignore the rest." She adds, "The most dramatic form of bias is out-and-out suppression of negative results."

You will rarely hear academia complain. Why? Because they are aboard the gravy train. Dr. Angell writes, "Columbia University, which patented the technology used in the manufacture of Epogen and Cerezyme, collected nearly $300 million in royalties" in seventeen years. Harvard is in just as deep: in its own Faustian dealings with the drug companies, "a Harvard hospital has a deal that gives Novartis rights to discoveries that lead to new cancer drugs (and) Merck is building a twelve-story research facility next door to Harvard Medical School." The result? "Bias is now rampant in drug trials. . . . (Pharmaceutical) industry-sponsored research was nearly four times as likely to be favorable to the company's product as NIH-sponsored research." *NIH-sponsored* means taxpayer funded research at the National Institutes of Health.

The pharmaceutical industry deploys an army of 88,000 energetic sales representatives, such that some physicians "may be visited by a dozen in one day." Dr. Angell says that drug companies see physicians as prescription delivery devices, and they are monitored accordingly. Drug reps "know exactly what a doctor prescribes before each visit" and "they can tell whether the visit paid off by seeing what the doctor does afterward." The pharmaceutical presence is everywhere you find a white coat and a beeper. "Drug reps are allowed to attend medical conferences, may be invited into operating and procedure rooms, and sometimes are even present when physicians examine patients in clinics or at the bedside. . . . It's a way to build business."

And what a business it is. Drug industry worldwide sales are approaching $500 billion per year, half of which are in North America. Profit margins are typically 20 percent, so high that, according to Dr. Angell, "the combined profits for the ten drug companies in the Fortune 500 were more than the profits for all the other 490 businesses put together."

years of medical school, is that in order to promote recovery of a condition, it is important to discover the cause. Well, of course! However this is a lesson not always remembered in a practicing physician's later years.

Let's examine the best possible scenario in conventional cancer treatment. When a specialist refers to conventional chemotherapy as being completely effective, what he means is that the patient was able to tolerate and survive the therapy and that the patient is in remission, which means the patient is now free of detectable disease. As we all know, the adverse effects of chemotherapy usually range from moderate to severe and can even be life-threatening. Achieving remission is great, but have we really dealt with the cause? Probably not. If there is a house infested with roaches, we can hire a professional licensed exterminator to come monthly and that will control the problem. However, if people in the house always leave food out in the kitchen, the insecticide and the traps will help, but only proper cleaning and handling of the food can deal with the cause of the problem. If you hire an exterminator and he starts shooting roaches with a flame thrower, and spraying acid all over, he might gain control of the roaches, but you will not be very comfortable . . . because he will destroy your house in the process. (Any similarity with any known medical practice is a mere coincidence!)

When solving any problem, you want to be rational and you want your health consultants to be rational. That sounds quite obvious, but in reality lots of people and clinicians go about trying to solve health problems with a general scheme that conforms to well-accepted standards. Such standards may not be entirely rational. They are profoundly affected by emotions, traditions, personal ambitions, politics, and money, which in the ultimate analysis are not the most beneficial influences for the patient.

THE LESSONS OF THE PAST

Now, let's look at what can be done about new ideas and new approaches. We will use the process of the "paradigm shift" in science to illustrate that, for centuries, there has been a resistance of the establishment to correct itself despite the evidence. For asserting that the sun, not the earth, was the center of the solar system, mathematician and astronomer Galileo Galilei (1564–1642) was severely criticized and threatened with punishment by the church, despite his outstanding discoveries. However, this phenomena was not limited to the sixteenth century, nor only to the topic of astronomy and its relation to religious beliefs.

Dr. Hugh D. Riordan (our mentor) wrote a series of books entitled *Medical Mavericks* in which he presented brief biographies of extraordinary clinicians and scientists who, through their detailed observation, careful analysis, clinical work, research, and documentation, advanced knowledge in the medical field in significant, and usually controversial, ways. The recurrent theme of these biographies was that even when good science was used to discover important knowledge, it was opposed, rejected, or ignored not on the basis of scientific merit but on the basis of prevailing opinions.[1] We want to summarize a few of these stories that revolve around the history of vitamin C, because by knowing history, we may avoid repeating the mistakes of an often intolerant past.

In 1747, Scottish naval surgeon James Lind discovered that something (now known to be vitamin C) in citrus foods prevented and cured scurvy. Lind provided some crew members with two oranges and one lemon per day, in addition to normal food rations, while others continued on their normal rations without citrus foods. (This experiment is considered to be the first example of a controlled clinical trial. Lind compared the results on two populations, where one known, new factor is applied to one group only, with all other factors remaining the same.) Lind published his work, *Treatise on the Scurvy*, in 1753. Since keeping fresh fruits on board sailing ships was difficult and inconvenient, some British naval officers had the "bright" idea of boiling their juice to produce a concentrate that allowed easy storage. That was very clever, except for one minuscule detail—they did not know that the substance that prevented scurvy (vitamin C) was destroyed by heat. Ship captains wrongly concluded that citrus fruits didn't work, because the concentrate failed to cure scurvy. It was like trying to put out a fire with a fire extinguisher that was empty.

After many years, this issue was reviewed, and finally in 1795 the British navy adopted lemons or limes as a standard ration item at sea. It took over forty years, and thousands of lives that succumbed to scurvy, before the work of Lind was properly appreciated, evaluated, and put into action to end unnecessary deaths. Shortly thereafter, British sailors came to be known as "limeys" due to their consumption of limes and lemons (and perhaps because "lemonies" does not sound nearly as good).

In another dramatic example from the mid-nineteenth century, the incidence of women dying after giving birth was nearly 20 percent. Hungarian physician Ignaz Philip Semmelweis (1818–1865) discovered in 1847 that doctors' hand-washing with chlorinated lime solutions reduced the incidence of fatal puerperal fever (severe systemic infection occurring during or soon after labor) to only about 1 percent. Instead of being honored, he was vilified for suggesting that all that mattered was cleanliness. At the time, the amount of blood on the physician's gown was a symbol of medical bravery. Some doctors would go directly from working on a cadaver at autopsy to deliver a baby . . . without washing their hands! Dr. Semmelweis was dismissed from his hospital post and had difficulty finding employment as a medical doctor. He had a tough life and was largely ignored, rejected, and ridiculed. Twenty years after his death, his doctrine was accepted by most physicians and a monument in his honor was erected in Budapest (better late than never!). Once again, Dr. Semmelweis's work correctly showed the way to protect a woman giving birth, but decades passed by and hundreds of women died because of failure to accept a concept that could be easily corroborated.

So, you might think that after all the advances in science during the last half of the twentieth century, today's medical science would be more rational. Well, not quite. Linus Pauling, Ph.D., two-time Nobel Prize laureate (Chemistry and Peace) is widely regarded as the premier chemist of the twentieth century. Dr. Pauling was a pioneer in the application of quantum mechanics to chemistry. He became an advocate of regular consumption of high doses of vitamin C and collaborated with Dr. Ewan Cameron on vitamin C and cancer research. In the late 1970s, they published the results of using intravenous and oral vitamin C at high doses with terminal cancer patients. The vitamin C–treated patients were found to have an average survival time about 300 days greater than that of the controls. These findings ignited many debates. How could the application of a simple, inexpensive vitamin yield such impressive results?

Soon after, a group from the Mayo Clinic, in Rochester, Minnesota, designed and conducted another trial to determine if they could get these results. Guess what happened? The Mayo Clinic group was unable to show a therapeutic benefit of high-dose vitamin C treatment in patients with advanced cancer. There is a reason why. In science, when you have two experiments testing a hypothesis and they give conflicting results, the first thing to do is look at the methodology (the way the trial was conducted). Well, the methodology was not the same. The Cameron and Pauling trial used *intravenous* administration for ten days and then they gave oral vitamin C, and the total daily amount was divided in several doses per day. *The Mayo Clinic group did not use intravenous administration and gave the entire daily amount in a single dose.* The medical establishment failed to consider these important methodological differences and decided that the matter was settled: vitamin C was declared "useless" in terminal cancer patients. Many oncologists still persist in this erroneous belief.

The original papers from these studies were published between 1976 and 1983 (see Appendix B). It wouldn't be long before somebody would shed more light on the apparently conflicting results. In 1992, Dr. Mark Levine and his group from the National Institutes of Health (NIH) published their findings about the absorption, mechanics, and disposition of ascorbic acid.[2] His findings allowed determination with scientific certainty that the method used in the trial by Cameron and Pauling exposed patients to substantially higher blood levels of vitamin C than the patients in the Mayo Clinic trial.

Common sense might also lead you to think that a difference in methodology would certainly cause different vitamin C blood levels. Then, of course, the medical establishment would have to want to reconsider their position and give Cameron and Pauling their due. If you think that, think again. When Dr. Levine published his findings in 1992, not much happened. The position of the oncological medical establishment on vitamin C and cancer was unchanged: after all, this issue was already settled at the Mayo Clinic!

Later in this book, we will continue the saga of vitamin C and cancer into the twenty-first century, where finally the light is beginning to be seen. For now, it's time to stop and recap. There is a recurrent theme in these lessons from the past: *discovery through good science is not enough to accept and integrate life-saving strategies into medicine.* One also needs a great deal of persistence.

CHOOSING YOUR HEALTH-CARE PROVIDER

You are an individual, not necessarily an "average person." You do not have the same needs as the previous patient in the oncologist's office. Each person has unique needs in terms of information, nutritional biochemistry, physical processes, finances, emotions, psychology, and spirituality. It is very important that you recognize your real needs and take charge of fulfilling them. If you do not, who will?

In particular, make sure that you feel comfortable with your health-care provider. You must be able to talk with your provider, and your doctor(s) must be able to talk *with* you not *at* you. The health-care provider must not only be knowledgeable, but be a sensitive, kind person who can fulfill your expectations in terms of availability, giving you enough time for your questions and treating you with respect. You are creating a support team in your healing process. If you are not receiving the support you need, express your needs and allow time for changes to occur. If that does not work, do not hesitate to fire someone who is not doing their job. Your needs must be fulfilled—it is your body, and your doctor works for you, not the other way around.

Since a "cancer" diagnosis and the treatment that follows may have important consequences in your life, it is always a good idea to have a second opinion. By getting a second opinion, you reduce the chances of diagnostic errors. You also allow yourself to compare therapeutic approaches in addition to experiencing the level of empathy with another practitioner.

Professional training and scientific education *should* provide the tools for doctors to be objective in evaluating available information and to facilitate the often difficult decisions with patients. It must be emphasized that the purpose of evaluation is to find out not only what the condition of the patient is, and what is the extent of the problem, but also defining cause(s). This will be discussed in more detail later. Such information is very important because *getting rid of a group of cancer cells or a tumor is different from regaining your health.*

THE NEED FOR A COMPREHENSIVE PLAN

Doctors learn a lot in medical school, but they do not learn everything. For example, there are many biological concepts about the nature of membrane receptors and about the biochemistry of inflammation and cell communication that are well documented in the scientific literature but are not part of most medical school training. There are also many valuable therapeutic tools that are not studied in medical school. This doesn't mean that these excluded bodies of knowledge are not important. Integration of knowledge into the medical school curriculum, or into your doctor's practice, takes time. Unfortunately, it often takes way too much time, and someone with a serious illness simply cannot wait.

We assert that optimum nutrition and scientific dietary supplementation should be part of every cancer treatment. Nutrition is not only preventive; it also has a powerful therapeutic potential. There are many conditions that develop precisely as a result of inadequate nutrition, or as a failure to recognize and satisfy an individual's higher nutrient needs. Nutrients can correct the underlying biochemical problems that allow the development of many diseases. Failure of clinicians to understand the value of scientific supplementation and nutrition can often lead to unnecessary suffering for many patients.

This is the realm of *orthomolecular medicine*, a term originated by Linus Pauling, which means "the right molecule in the right place." *Orthomolecular medicine restores the optimum environment of the body by correcting imbalances or deficiencies based on individual biochemistry.* In conventional medicine, the power of nutrition and scientific high-dose nutrient supplementation is generally underestimated as part of the treatment of most chronic diseases, especially cancer. The main reasons for this neglect is related to nutrition's gradual (instead of immediate) effect upon disease; to institutional resistance to change; to our "magic bullet" wishful thinking in regard to medicine; to the counterforce of aggressive drug marketing; and to the lack of emphasis in this area in medical education. Dr. Riordan often said, "*Orthomolecular* is not the answer to any question posed in medical school."

When a patient visits a clinician, he or she usually expects to see an expert who, after a review of the case, would be capable of selecting the most suitable treatment plan for the condition. This plan should be a comprehensive one that improves the overall health and well-being of the patient. However, very often for a specialist in oncology, the therapeutic approaches offered are mainly limited to surgery, radiation, and chemotherapy. Such limitation reminds us of the proverb "When you are holding a hammer, everything resembles a nail."

While these therapeutic strategies may have value in certain patients, keep in mind that in the treatment of any disease, it is of utmost importance to correct the cause of the problem. Surgery removes a tumor without addressing what formed it in the first place. We have never seen a case of cancer caused by a deficiency of radiation or chemotherapy. So, if you want comprehensive treatment, it is imperative to look at causes in every individual case.

If you need help finding a natural healing–oriented (naturopathic or orthomolecular) physician, we have some suggestions:

- First, try an Internet search engine (such as Google).This is one of the easiest and fastest ways to search far and wide.

- Health food stores are sometimes helpful referral sources, as may be a health magazine or a look through the telephone directory.

- Ask your friends or ask members of a patients' support group.

- Inquiring at your local public library can be especially productive. If you are not confident in your searching, ask a librarian for assistance. We have found librarians to be extremely helpful, with only the rarest of exceptions. If by chance you meet an unsympathetic librarian, just try a different library. The authors of this book all have doctorates, and we still ask librarians for assistance. Why? Because they are so expert at finding information.

- You can request a list of orthomolecular (nutritional medicine) practitioners near where you live by contacting Steven Carter, managing editor of the *Journal of Orthomolecular Medicine* (e-mail: scarter@ orthomed.org). There may be a requested fee for this.

PERSONAL LOSSES FROM CANCER

"I have cancer. What should I do?" We know how you feel. We've been there. This is not your average book about cancer. We do not come to this subject—cancer—simply as practitioners. We also have had personal experiences with this potentially devastating disease.

Michael's Story

In 1978, I was in high school and interested in science, boxing, and basketball (not necessarily in that order). I was fascinated with biology and thinking of solving the impossible: death and cancer. I was raised by my maternal grandparents, who had jumped onto a transatlantic immigrant ship with a dollar in their pockets during the Great Depression years. My grandfather landed a job as a janitor at the Con Edison Company in New York; he worked his way up and retired as an assistant engineer. My grandmother worked as a cook in Brooklyn.

In 1979, I read an article by Linus Pauling entitled "Ascorbic Acid and Cancer."[3] This article totally enticed and mesmerized me. A vitamin helping fight a disease that nobody really understands? Wait a minute: this is really something, I thought. I can see myself studying this as a career. So, I decided to write a paper about this for my science class.

A couple weeks later, my grandfather was diagnosed with liver cancer. The doctor told my grandmother that the disease was pretty far advanced and there was nothing he could do. I told her, we can put him on intravenous vitamin C (10,000 milligrams per day). I went home and searched for my papers and decided to show them to the doctor. He was a very kind and open-minded man and, knowing the disease was in a terminal stage, he agreed to try the vitamin C. We gave him about 4 or 5 doses and his pain and discomfort were substantially alleviated (to the doctor's amazement). My grandfather eventually died a couple months later, a hard hit for me and my grandmother.

My second encounter with cancer came when I was starting my doctoral studies in nutrition and biochemistry at Michigan State University. While I was there studying fats and cancer, my grandmother was diagnosed with metastasized colon cancer. I was having difficulty with a biochemistry class and was not able to travel to see her. We did give her some intravenous vitamin C (10 grams, twice a week) and it helped a bit. (I now think more C would have done more.) A couple of months later, she passed away. I went to the basement of the library and cried. But after this, I vowed to fight cancer until I could find something important in understanding and conquering it.

A third encounter with cancer came when my mother was diagnosed with melanoma. This event really surprised me since my mother had fairly dark skin. We tried intravenous vitamin C (15 grams, two times a week) and it definitely enhanced her quality of life, but eventually she, too, died of the disease.

I am telling you this to let you know that fighting cancer is something very personal for me. Cancer has taken three of the most important people in my life.

Jorge's Story

When my father died of cancer, I was four years old, and that was my first experience with death. Being so young, I did not realize what was going on. This loss had an important impact in my life in many ways. For one thing, it put pressure on my mother to become a provider, and consequently my grandmother had a lot of responsibility in raising me and my brother. My mother worked with three of her brothers in my grandfather's pharmacy. My grandfather was a well respected pharmacist, and the family pharmacy started operations in San Juan, Puerto Rico, back in 1947. For the first few decades, there was a lot of pharmaceutical compounding as well as the use of natural substances. As my grandfather reached his late seventies, he relied more on my mother and my uncle Herbert to take charge of the business.

Herbert was the pharmacist I most remember and he became my role model as he was the closest I had to a father. Watching him gave me a great deal of inspiration to become what I am today. He was very hard working, and this came from his strong commitment to improve the health-care system and take care of people through his profession. I learned from him the importance of developing a worthy vision of the future. My mother was very hard working also. Making sure that the pharmacy would provide truly good service was always her foremost concern. As a kid, I used go to the pharmacy to read the comic books. Even though my conscious mind was on my reading, I was aware of everything that was happening there. With time, I would learn enough to start helping the pharmacist and soon I was able to anticipate most of the professional recommendations.

One of the most important experiences that molded my values and way of thinking was observing many people suffering multiple chronic conditions that required multiple medications. What got my attention was that many of these people were sick *despite* following the conventional wisdom in terms of medical recommendations. I saw patients in their fifties and sixties getting ten or twelve different medications, paying large amounts of money, and still having a poor quality of life. I thought they must be doing something wrong (or not doing something right) that was causing their health problems. Perhaps drugs could help somewhat in maintenance, but not quite enough to truly cure. Reflecting on these observations, I concluded that I wanted to learn how to live a healthy life so that I could avoid most of these diseases and, like my grandparents, reach old age being healthy, happy, mentally sharp, and vigorous.

When I started college, I decided to study pharmacy. At that time, most pharmacy programs offered a professional bachelor's degree.

During my second year of the program, I realized I wanted a more in-depth education and decided to pursue a doctoral degree in pharmacy. After being accepted in several programs, I selected the Philadelphia College of Pharmacy and Sciences (now Philadelphia University of the Sciences), one of the best schools of pharmacy. In Philadelphia, I met Miriam, who was doing research at Temple University, and we married just before my graduation.

After completing my doctoral degree and postdoctoral training, we moved back to Puerto Rico so that I could start my new job as an assistant professor in the School of Pharmacy at the University of Puerto Rico Medical Sciences Campus. Three years later, my wife gave birth to our second child. It was a time of great happiness, but shortly after we received terrible news. Miriam had been dealing with a problem in one of her breasts in the later stages of her pregnancy. A few months after she gave birth, it turned out that the problem was a very aggressive, locally advanced cancer.

It was a very distressing and confusing time in our lives. As most people would do, we sought for the most well-respected authorities. After initial evaluation, our oncologist recommended aggressive chemotherapy. He specifically warned us not to use vitamins and other antioxidants as they could protect the cancer cells from chemotherapy. He also recommended evaluation for a possible bone marrow transplant. During that time (mid-1990s), it was thought that the higher the dose of the chemotherapeutic agent, the higher the chance of killing all cancer cells. The problem with this strategy is that the therapy is so toxic that it kills blood cells and the patient needs extraordinary medical measures to protect him or her from life-threatening infections and anemia until they can recover. Another problem is that chemotherapy weakens the immune system, which is a critical system for cancer control.

When friends and family members heard the bad news, they were very supportive and many offered recommendations that had helped or supposedly saved the life of someone they knew. Miriam and I discussed the situation and she agreed that I should study the matter and get the most reliable information to empower us to make the wisest decisions. She did not have much of a response to the conventional treatment; indeed, it made her feel weaker. She was evaluated in Memorial Sloan-

Kettering Cancer Center as a candidate for a bone marrow transplant. Believe it or not, that treatment was not covered by the medical insurance at that time, and the cost was around $400,000. It was quite stressful to have the specialists recommending a treatment that medical insurance would not pay for and that was utterly beyond our financial abilities.

Because of my academic position, I had access to more information than most people and at least I could find out the details as to how it was supposed to work. I thought that the oncologist should provide patients with alternatives to *all* treatment plans, so that he would give every patient a better chance to access treatment. I felt abandoned by my medical insurance company when I most needed it. In addition, I found studies that contradicted what the oncologist told me about the concurrent use of chemotherapy and the effectiveness of some vitamins and nutrients. There were reports stating that some nutrients improve the response while decreasing toxicity of chemotherapy. But none of our doctors would address this issue.

I found a bone marrow transplant protocol for breast cancer sponsored by the National Cancer Institute (NCI) and Miriam qualified. She participated and received the bone marrow transplant. Little did I know that this experience would be more a learning experience for me than a healing experience for Miriam. While there, I read that there was an explosion in the use of alternative medicine and there was now an office of Complementary and Alternative Medicine (CAM) in the NIH. The most prestigious medical schools were now beginning to include CAM in their curriculum. These trends stimulated my interest in the area in an irreversible way.

Six months after the transplant, Miriam was doing much worse. She felt weaker and had several complications. Her follow-up computerized tomography (CT) scans showed that tumors had now spread all over the place. Needless to say, I had a very hard time when she passed away. I spent much time reflecting on all that happened and revising the goals of my life. I would do everything I could to be the healthiest that I could be so that my children would not lose their father. I also wanted to contribute to the development of more effective, less toxic cancer therapies.

Andrew's Story

I have been lucky. Although my grandparents, parents, and many other relatives are long gone, few have died from cancer. In her advanced years, my mother had a small breast tumor that was malignant but evidently not metastasized. They took it out and gave her radiation, and that was the end of that. She died years later, but not from cancer. Her father, a heavy smoker, died of lung cancer when I was two years old. Having never known him, I never knew the loss, but my mother sure did. After hearing my mother relate the whole grim story, I never wanted to try a single cigarette. I still don't.

The worst personal cancer losses for me were my two cousins. One, a lovely young woman who relentlessly chased me around the house when we were kids, was killed in her early thirties by brain cancer. The other cousin, a very talented stage performer, contracted cancer very suddenly and died at fifty-one. I still miss them both.

YOUR SUPPORT NETWORK

In spite of the personal losses we have suffered, we have learned that cancer is never a death sentence. Cancer is an opportunity to live, to examine your true values and see if you are living according to your beliefs, to reflect on whether or not you are doing what matters the most. Are you giving something of yourself to make this world better? Are you giving all the love and gratitude you can give? Have you forgiven that someone who has done you wrong? We have learned that you need to be in touch with your feelings and be empowered with knowledge and self-esteem in order to begin the healing journey.

Life is most certainly a journey. The question is, *what kind* of a journey will it be for you? What matters most is not the ultimate destination, but to rather enjoy the ride and the wonderful scenes along the way. Help everybody you can to make that journey better, comfortable, easier, and happy. We want to share with you what has made the life of many people so much better.

Having said that, we think patients with a recent diagnosis of cancer should acknowledge that this can be one of the most stressful and challenging times in their life. Therefore, it is important to create a support group that includes family and friends that can contribute to make this time more bearable. Close friends and relatives must be there to listen and support your emotional as well as other needs, such as appropriate food, daily household chores, and other special considerations, such as reasonable adaptations to conditions at work.

Create a daily routine that is uplifting to your spirit that includes laughter, exercise, meditation or prayer, and contact with nature. Select and seek out your ideal physical, emotional, and social environment. As you develop an awareness of what is good for you and what is not, seek environments that are comfortable for you and that give you support and energy, and avoid environments that drain you. This is a time for reflection, inspiration, and transformation. Survivors are people who are empowered to make decisions and take command. Survivors are motivated by hope and a vision of their future that is full of passion. When that energy is present, there is a powerful message of healing from the mind and spirit to the body.

This is just an opening stance; we will provide many more specific treatment options as the book unfolds.

A COMPREHENSIVE APPROACH TO CANCER

People die from cancer every day, in all families, everywhere. There is no comfort in that statement. How do we make sense of it? It is scary and confusing. Sometimes we feel that, if all the world's a stage, then we do not know our lines. Here we are, on the stage of life, surrounded with everybody else who seems to know what they are doing. Well, they don't. They are winging it, perhaps just like you. Good faith leads cancer patients to their oncologists and their oncologists' good faith leads them to order surgery, radiation, and chemotherapy. These are often helpful, but they are almost as often not helpful. Either way, they are not enough. To have the best chance of beating cancer, we also need to have optimal nutrition and lifestyle changes.

What would we do if we had cancer? We'd follow the program in this book:

- Positive psychological/spiritual empowerment
- Proper nutrition
- Supplementation
- Effective, nontoxic therapies
- Detoxification
- Exercise
- Relaxation

I (Andrew) also would immediately start the Gerson nutritional therapy (Chapter 3), based on fresh vegetable juices and organic whole foods. And, I would most assuredly follow Dr. Riordan's protocol and receive intravenous vitamin C, followed by high oral maintenance doses. We will discuss that later in this book. It is all good news! In fact, it is so good that I am following much of this comprehensive program now just for prevention, because I do not want to have to follow it later for treatment. I eat right and take handfuls of vitamins several times every day. Works for me; my doctor says I'm in great shape and I make her job easy. That's the idea.

As a professional consultant, I personally have seen what nutrition can do for a terminally ill cancer patient. I have been called upon to help in a couple of high-profile but last minute cases. One patient was a well-known sports figure who was given just months to live and was not happy about it, as he was still in his fifties. He asked what his best shot would be for inoperable, untreatable metastasized cancer. I told him: aggressive nutritional therapy involving dietary changes and supplements. He did it, not in its entirety, but with enthusiasm—and he lived considerably longer than he was expected to. But what really impressed me was the dramatic improvement in his energy level: from fatigue and weakness, he went instantly to a vibrant life, commencing from the very week he started the program. He maintained a more-than-full schedule for so long that even people who knew he was sick forgot about it. Years later, people who never knew of my involvement in the matter would bring up his name, invariably recalling how active he was and how good he looked until, almost as a surprise, he died.

I saw a similar level of success with a prominent New York businessman, the owner of a chain of stores who was afflicted with untreatable liver cancer. He began to do much, but by no means all, of the program, and was subsequently able to extensively travel the world with his family. He lived years longer than expected, with a high quality of life confirmed by all who saw him.

Neither of these patients followed the diet and supplement program completely. It is an admittedly tough sell, even to a person with a terminal diagnosis. Labor-intensive as any lifestyle change is, this approach has been seen to significantly improve both quality of life and length of life in cancer patients. Many people have been completely cured. One was a schoolteacher and friend of mine with breast cancer. She drank the juices and took vitamins. She also had conventional therapy, but none of the common side effects: nausea, hair loss, appetite loss, and radiation burning. She has kept in touch occasionally over the decades and is alive today.

For a presumed-terminal patient, any improvement at all is cause for celebration. Slowing the rate of decline is improvement. Stabilization is better. Some recovery is better still. Cure is, of course, the best. Improved length of life is a major goal, but improved quality of life is the most important of all.

You might well wonder, since presumably I learned something useful about how to fight cancer, why two of my cousins still died from it. From what I've seen, it is your own family members that may need information the most and accept it the least. If you are peeved because your relations, who you'd think should know better, don't listen to your healthy advice, here is some tart advice from my grandmother to give them: "Do as you like," she used to say. "You will anyway."

There are two kinds of patients. Those who will listen politely, nod their head, and do nothing; and those who will be discouraged, skeptical, and a little bit desperate, and who are actually more likely to go for it. Quoting Michael Ash, M.D., of Cornwall, England: "All my patients die. The question is, When?" It's not about whether you got sick; it's about how you get well, and how long you stay that way. Perhaps the best way I have found to deal with all this is to take a "buffet" approach: put the information in plain view and let them take all, some, or none, as they will.

I hope you will take all of it.

A LITTLE MOTIVATION

Back in the 1930s, humorist Will Rogers was very interested in the new and growing aviation industry. At a meeting he was attending, corporate big shots were discussing the possibility of issuing parachutes to passengers for use in case of emergency. They mentioned that if parachutes were available, most passengers would not be able to put them on in time, and those that did might not have time or room to get to an exit. They concluded that of the dozen or so passengers on a flight, probably only one would be saved. Rogers leaned back in his chair, put his boots up on the conference table, tipped his hat down over his eyes, and said: "But wouldn't *he* be just tickled."

Naysayers are fond of pointing out that natural healing methods do not always work on everybody. But they don't have to: they only have to work on you, or one of your family, to make the biggest possible difference. Medical doctors generally fight disease with one hand tied behind their backs. This is because they arrogantly assume that if they don't know it, it isn't knowable or worth knowing. Baloney. Aggressive use of vitamins and radical diet revision *do* have their place in the science of therapeutics.

Linus Pauling estimated that disease and mortality could be reduced by at least 25 percent if people took large daily quantities of essential vitamins. Let's say he was way off, and the improvement was only 1 percent. Since upwards of 2 million Americans die each year, a 1 percent improvement would save 20,000 people; if Dr. Pauling was right, 500,000 people.

So be a health nut, and show the world. You really do make a difference, and don't you forget it! In the sixties, one slogan was "What if they gave a war, and nobody came?" Enough individual actions should add up to peace. Well, what if each person eats right, exercises, eradicates their bad habits, and starts taking vitamins? Might our new slogan be: "What if they gave everybody health insurance, and nobody needed it?" The result would be nothing less than total national health, gained one person at a time.

Oddly enough, it may be that we've had trouble seeing the trees because of the forest. Health care is such an enormous issue that we tend to bite off more than we can chew. Getting a nation to be healthy is a tall order. To think we can ever gain national health by refinancing the same old disease model is ludicrous. As difficult as it truly is to change our own personal habits, it remains the only sure method to gain our own health and to positively influence another person to do the same. In the end, this project really comes down to the education and motivation in just one person's health behavior—yours.

Today, Americans have real health options but are largely unaware of the safety, the scientific validity, and the real curative power of simple nutrients. It is regrettable that often patients are never informed that they even have choices, such as nutritional supplements, whole-foods diet, or fresh raw vegetable juices, and that these alternatives can really work. This can and must change. We must advocate, and personally choose, that less-traveled route if it will lead us to health.

Patient Words to Help Patients Be More Patient

- Daily health progress may fluctuate or plateau; relax and stay with it. Sometimes it is useful to be reminded that we are not in a hurry. After all, how long did it take to get in this condition in the first place?

- People may lose confidence in their ability to break a habit or to get better. They may quit and not return. But you don't have to do everything all at once. We'd rather you do most of what is suggested in this book for a year than do all of it for a week.

- Each patient needs to learn *not* to be a patient, but rather to be their own doctor. On the road to self-reliance, friend and family support is nice to have, but truth be told, you cannot always count on it.

WHAT THIS BOOK IS ABOUT

What would we, personally, do if we had cancer? This book will answer that question. Because we were trained as scientists, our book will next be offering you scientific evidence that alternative cancer therapies are effective. But there is more to it than that. When a scientist goes home at the end of the day, he is a parent or husband like anyone else. Therefore, we will also offer something else: our humanity. Our message to you is based on a quest that was ignited by passion and compassion: a passion for the discovery and dissemination of knowledge, and compassion to fellow human beings suffering from cancer. These twin motivators have been greatly amplified by our own personal losses. It is rare to find a family or a person who has not lost someone to cancer. This book is inspired by the love of people who are not physically among us anymore but whose lives taught us many important lessons.

CHAPTER 2

Knowing the Enemy

"Do not follow where the path may lead.
Go instead where there is no path and leave a trail."
—ANONYMOUS

Cancer may be humanity's most feared disease. It is certainly one of the most complex. If there were a sure cure for cancer, you would have heard about it already, and this book would be two pages long. But cancer persists, even with all the efforts of science and the expenditure of billions of research dollars over decades. Even experts do not agree. No wonder persons with cancer are so often confused, and so often scared.

THE CANCER PROCESS

Your body contains trillions of cells. Within each cell, there is a central part known as the nucleus, wherein lies the key to life itself—an immensely long, twisted ladder–shaped molecule of deoxyribonucleic acid (DNA). DNA contains the instructions (genes) that each cell needs to make its vital proteins as well as to replicate itself. Abnormal changes in a cell's DNA are called mutations. These mutations can be lethal and the cell will die, or it may continue to divide uncontrolled into a mass called a tumor.

Mutations are usually associated with exposure to radiation, heavy metals, and other toxic substances. However, there are many other factors related to lifestyle that can determine risks of developing cancer.

Stress, poor food choices, and other bad habits can alter physiology and provide the proper environment for malignant transformation at the cellular level. Malignant transformation may occur when DNA expression is influenced by biochemical changes that affect cell metabolism and energy.

There are two types of tumors, benign and malignant. Benign tumors are not cancerous because the cells, although disturbed, are still more or less normal. Most benign tumors do not pose a threat to life; cells from a benign tumor do not spread to other parts of the body. Malignant tumors are composed of cancerous cells. These cells are far from normal, and they can invade and damage nearby tissues and organs.

Embryonic Development and Carcinogenesis

After fertilization, early embryonic cells receive the genetic instruction to multiply rapidly. There is a point at which the genetic instructions change after a certain number of cell divisions so that some cells start producing specific proteins. This process is called differentiation.

The embryonic developmental process goes from the very simple and primitive to the very specialized and complex. In contrast, in the development of cancer (carcinogenesis), this process is reversed: you start with cells in a mature, specialized tissue that, at a certain point, are forced to go back to the original, more primitive state (cell division without differentiation). The importance of understanding this contrast between both processes (embryonic development and carcinogenesis) is that if you modulate the biochemical environment, you may be able to reverse this malignant process. Normal cells in a differentiated tissue can be deranged when exposed to certain adverse conditions (radiation, heavy metals, and other toxic substances), producing alterations in gene expression that can reverse differentiation and promote the primitive survival state of fast cell division without differentiation. This is how tumors develop. Correcting the biochemical environment can direct cell physiology to return to its normal path toward the differentiated, nonmalignant state.

Steps in Cancer Development

There are three key steps in cancer development: initiation, promotion, and progression. Some kind of a change in a cell, tissue, or organ is necessary to begin the carcinogenic process. Such a change may be caused by exposure to a cancer-causing agent (carcinogen). This is called *initiation*. Initiation may or may not be sufficient to result in cancer. There is a second necessary step, called *promotion*. Promotion is when initiated cells actually start to proliferate. We all know what *progression* is: cancerous cells continue to grow and extend out into normal cells.

BIOENERGETICS THEORY OF CARCINOGENESIS

We believe that the altered metabolism of tumor cells can provide a target for nontoxic, effective cancer therapy. Normal cells tend to degenerate when their oxygen (aerobic) respiration is reduced or impaired. When this occurs, the cells, in an effort to survive this hostile environment, gradually change their metabolic energy-producing process to fermentation (sugar fermentation) in order to fulfill their energy needs. This is an inefficient, anaerobic (without oxygen) process, although it is capable of sustaining life. This primitive metabolic process is common to non-differentiated cells, such as cancer cells. The end product of fermentation is lactic acid instead of carbon dioxide gas. This end product acidifies the cell's environment, perpetuating this inefficient metabolic shift. As this process continues, biochemical parameters change and these cells physically resemble primitive forms very similar to embryonic cells.

This process is called de-differentiation, a reversion of specialized cells to a more generalized or primitive form often as a preliminary to major physiological change. As the cells go through this de-differentiation process, they look and behave like primitive cells. These primitive cells are capable of uncontrolled division and growth, and this uncontrolled growth is what we know as cancer.

Cancer cells rely on fermentation for energy and, as mentioned earlier, fermentation is a very inefficient process (it produces two units of adenosine triphosphate or ATP while respiration produces 36–38 ATP units) and demands more energy than the body can afford. So, the body, in order to survive, converts lactic acid back to sugar (glucose) by the Cori cycle. This process is very expensive in terms of energy and the body wastes away. This is called cachexia, which leads eventually to death, usually either by pneumonia or heart failure.

It has been demonstrated that the intermittent withholding of oxygen from a cell can transform it into a cancer cell. So, high blood viscosity, reduced circulation, and low oxygen supply, in addition to nutritional or chemical impairment to the mitochondria (oxygen respiratory organelle), can promote carcinogenesis. In fact, we believe that mitochondrial damage, if pronounced enough, can initiate the cancer process itself.

An increased glucose consumption rate has been observed in malignant cells. Otto Warburg (1883–1970), a German physician-scientist and Nobel laureate, postulated that when the respiratory process of cells is impaired, the transformation of normal cells to malignant cells is due to defects in the aerobic respiratory pathway. This important discovery happened in the 1920s. In other words, cancer seems to have its root in the cell's energy-producing system.

Another Nobel Prize winner, Hungarian physician-scientist Albert Szent-Györgyi (1893–1986) also viewed cancer as originating from the cell's energy-producing system. He observed that insufficient availability of oxygen was present in malignancy. Oxygen itself has an inhibitory action on malignant cell growth by interfering with anaerobic respiration, the main energy source of the malignant cells (fermentation and lactic acid production). Interestingly, during cell differentiation (where the cell energy level is very high), there is an increase in cellular production of oxidative molecules that appear to provide a physiological stimulation for changes in gene expression, which may lead to a terminal differentiated state. This differentiated state overcomes malignancy. What we are saying here is that malignant tissue grows in the absence of oxygen and utilizes anaerobic (without oxygen) energy production, which reduces the production of oxidative species (free radicals) that may control cell division and differentiation, and increases the use of the sugar (glucose) fermentation process and the production of lactic acid, which favor the malignant environment.

The failure to maintain high ATP production, which is the primary and most effective form of cellular energy, may be a consequence of inactivation of key enzymes, especially those related to the Krebs cycle (enzyme reactions that help the cell utilize oxygen) and the electron transport system. Also, this might be due to a deficiency of cofactors (vitamins, minerals, nutrient molecules) needed by these important enzymes. A distorted mitochondrial function may result (the mitochondria are the energy factories of the cell). This could be highly suggestive of an important, yet obviated, mitochondrial involvement in the carcinogenic process.

German physician Max Gerson divided the cancer process into two main components, the general component and the local component. The general component comprises mainly the deterioration of the essential organs of the digestive tract, especially the liver. The damage is done by a daily poisoning brought about by our modern lifestyle (mainly bad dietary habits and toxin exposure). The subsequent change in cells from normal to primitive embryonic-like form by means of fermentation (the local component) was ascribed to an inadequacy of oxidizing enzymes, a potassium shortage, and an excess of sodium. The essential components of mitochondrial cell respiration are light-absorbing molecules that react to frequencies from the near ultraviolet band down to the yellow/orange spectral range of visible light.

Our physiological–biochemical state can be affected by lack of nutrients, unbalanced electrolytes, and the presence of toxins. This flow of electrons in the organs of respiration gives rise to a pulsating electromagnetic field which, activated by enzymes, may lead to an energy transfer to the body. This chemical–physical process is highly susceptible to any of the previously mentioned disturbances.

To summarize:

- Cancer is an anaerobic disease.
- Cancer uses fermentation of sugar for energy.
- Cancer accumulates lactic acid.

- Cancer is associated with lack of oxygen.

- Cancer is associated with deficiency of metabolic intermediate cofactors.

- Cancer can be associated with mitochondrial dysfunction.

- Cancer seems to be a disrupted energy disease.

HOW CANCER PROGRESSES

Let's take a quick look at how cancer runs its course. Understanding this aspect of the disease will help you understand why diet and additional nutritional support are so important in cancer therapy. The complexity of multicellular organisms requires an intricate mechanism to ensure that each gene is expressed at the right time and at the right place. After the sperm fertilizes the ovum, rapid cellular division begins without differentiation. This continues until a critical mass is achieved. Once this occurs, differentiation starts. Three germinal layers (endoderm, mesoderm, and ectoderm) are formed from which all tissues of the body arise. This is achieved by the regulated process of gene expression, which is controlled by several complex molecular signals. We believe this process is partly controlled by the mitochondria (more on this later). Erroneous expression of certain genes may cause cancers.

To understand the development of malignancy, we should take a look at the regulation of gene expression. There are segments of the DNA known as proto-oncogenes that are responsible for cell growth and activity. They regulate the way a cell develops and divides, and they also keep the order in the steps of the cell cycle. The proto-oncogenes are involved in early embryogenesis, where cell division occurs without differentiation. When proto-oncogenes mutate and convert into oncogenes, they order the cells to divide rapidly without differentiation, producing a tumor.

Tumor cells produce proteins that generate the growth of new blood vessels, which will bring more blood and nutrients to nourish the tumor. As the tumor grows, it may compress and harm organs and cause dysfunction. Cancer cells sometimes spread to new sites by a process called metastasis.

Cancer is classified by its appearance under a microscope as well as by the part of the body in which it primarily developed:

• Carcinoma: Malignant tumor that began in the lining layer (epithelial cells) of organs. Approximately 80 percent of all cancers are carcinomas.

• Sarcoma: Malignant tumors growing from connective tissue such as cartilage, fat, muscle, or bone.

• Leukemias: Cancers involving the blood and blood-forming organs (bone marrow, lymphatic system, and spleen).

• Lymphoma: Cancers involving the lymphatic system.

GERM THEORY VS. TERRAIN THEORY

Now, we'll take a closer look at the germ and terrain theories in order to explain what we want to accomplish in cancer treatment and why.

The germ theory of disease proposes that microbes are the main cause of many diseases. It was popularized by the French scientist Louis Pasteur (1822–1895). In order to get well, you need to identify and then kill whatever germ made you sick. The tools generally employed are drugs (antibiotics). Prevention includes the use of vaccines as well as drugs, which supposedly work by keeping germs at bay.

Just prior to the time when Pasteur began promoting the germ theory, Claude Bernard (1813–1878) was proposing the idea that the overall condition of the body is what determines the susceptibility to disease. Disease occurred when the "terrain" (body) conditions are deteriorated. A contemporary of Bernard, Antoine Béchamp (1816–1908), a scholar and medical doctor, further developed the terrain theory of health and disease. Disease occurs when metabolic processes are impaired causing a deleterious effect on biological function. When the metabolism is faulty, a lack in certain nutrients may promote excess oxidation and DNA damage. This DNA damage in certain areas can promote the needed metabolic changes to favor cell proliferation. If in addition to this, the immune system is not working properly, it will fail to control and neutralize abnormal cell growth. Thus, the body is in effect a mini-ecosystem, or a biological terrain in which a number of factors determine whether we stay healthy or become ill.

Biological Terrain

A healthy or diseased biological terrain is determined primarily by four things:

- Acid/alkaline balance (pH)

- Electric/magnetic charge (negative or positive)

- Level of poisoning (toxicity)

- Nutritional status

Critical symptoms of diseased terrain include low oxygen, stoppage of movement or stagnation in the body fluids between cells, and loss of electrical charge on the surface of cells. Disease seems to be the consequences of physiological imbalances, and the cellular universe operates by keeping opposites in balance. So, health is achieved by balancing the biological systems. If you want to see a rough comparison of what's happening in a sick body, try not cleaning your house for about a year. In that environment, all kinds of small "guests" will come out to take up residence with you. Similarly, wrong eating habits and risky lifestyles (such as smoking) increase damage of our inner bio-environment (terrain).

Our terrain becomes overly acidic, paving the way for disease. Normal blood pH is slightly alkaline between 7.35 and 7.45. However, the pH in the tissues may vary due to local conditions related to lifestyle factors (for example, diet). The excess acidity occurs due to dietary factors such as high intake of refined carbohydrates, saturated fats, and excess protein and deficiencies in critical nutrients. Other factors include poor oxygenation, the use of certain medications, obesity, and strong and sustained emotional stress. Excess acid in the tissues decreases the ability of the body to respond to biological stress and perform tissue repair.

Several critical biological enzymes that have important functions in

the immune system, neurological system, tissue repair, and energy production have optimal activity within a slightly alkaline environment.
When tissues are overly acidic, all these functions decrease and therefore are less effective.

The key to the development of disease lies in the condition of your
terrain. Is it in balance or will it support the development of disease?
Once the imbalance gets going, it becomes a vicious cycle. Poor digestion may occur and food may be sitting for too long in the gut, putre-
fying and decaying. In the early stages of this imbalance, the symptoms
may not be very intense and are frequently treated (manipulated) with
drugs. They include such things as skin eruptions, headaches, allergies,
and sinus problems. As things get further out of balance, more serious
conditions arise, such as weakened glands and organs, and body systems
start to deteriorate. These may include the thyroid, adrenal glands, and
the liver.

Unfortunately, symptom manipulation plays a major role in creating
an even worse disease condition later, but most people don't realize this
when they go for a quick medical fix. Even most doctors are not aware
of it. The most common medical approach is the use of aggressive
chemical therapy over a more natural, less aggressive, user-friendly
treatment. To put it more starkly, more poisons over food. In other
words, *we are feeding people poisons (drugs) trying to attack the consequences
of starvation (nutrient deficiency).*

To summarize, in the initial stages of human development after con-
ception, when our bodies are forming, we have cells that reproduce
rapidly without differentiation. This is a normal and needed process.
There are biological mechanisms that act to control cell growth and
induce differentiation. Genes are molecules of information that direct
these processes with the help of the mitochondria (energy provider).
At the same time, gene expression depends on and is influenced by biochemical signals provided by the cellular environment. The body has
the capacity to compensate biochemical derangements to some extent,
but there is a limit. When lack of certain nutrients, acidic environment, and toxins persist in the body, that limit is surpassed and damage occurs. That is the proper biological terrain for cancer to develop.

There are terrains (bodies) more susceptible than others due to specific genetic makeup (biochemical individuality) and lifestyle choices of each person. However, regardless of the genetic makeup, the terrain can be improved and that is the best way to keep the enemy away.

A NEW DIRECTION IN CANCER RESEARCH

Michael and I (Jorge) became friends as students at the Medical Sciences Campus of the University of Puerto Rico. We lost contact upon graduation, but several years later we met again as faculty members at the same campus. Michael liked my idea of a new interdisciplinary course in complementary and alternative medicine, and I was interested in his cancer research ideas. We started working together and collaborated on many research manuscripts for publication. Eventually, we started giving continuing medical education courses and created an education and research initiative called the Institute of Biochemical Medicine of Puerto Rico (InBioMed) and its main research project was called RECNAC II. "RECNAC" is *cancer* written backwards. After all, the goal is to reduce cancer! It is a continuation of Dr. Hugh D. Riordan's original RECNAC project at the Center for the Improvement of Human Functioning, in Wichita, Kansas. Dr. Riordan became our mentor and we established a collaboration with the center he founded, and this collaboration has led to more research and publications throughout the years (see Appendix C).

At the first Cancer Treatment Center Conference in 1987, I (Michael) met Neil H. Riordan, who was working with his father, Hugh, at the center. We met in the lobby of the hotel where we were staying around 9 P.M. and we ended up talking about our ideas and theories of cancer until 2:30 A.M. The next day, he invited me to Wichita and we immediately became collaborators. Later, in 1992, I attended a Linus Pauling talk. I had the chance to meet, chat, and express my ideas about cancer to two-time Nobel Prize winner Dr. Pauling. I told him about my idea of oxidation-reduction, energy, mitochondria, and their relation to cancer. At the end of the conversation, he said, "Young man, I am very happy because orthomolecular medicine is in good hands. Keep up the good work." This comment greatly inspired my life!

In 1999, during a FASEB (Federation of American Societies of Experimental Biology) conference on antioxidants in Vermont, I had the chance to talk to Dr. Mark Levine of the National Institutes of Health (NIH). He's been a principal researcher working with oral vitamin C pharmacokinetics. I mentioned to him that during my visit to the Center for the Improvement of Human Functioning, it was observed that in patients receiving 15 grams of intravenous vitamin C cancer cannot be traced in the serum. He said that was not possible. Dr. James A. Jackson, director of the clinical laboratory of the center, was present there and Dr. Levine was then invited to Wichita. This visit sparked a new era in cancer research. Dr. Levine has been very active in researching the pharmacokinetics of high-dose intravenous vitamin C and its effect on cancer.

- We published a study in 2002 in which we demonstrated an in vitro inhibiting effect of vitamin C on breast cancer cells.[1]

- In 2005, Dr. Levine and his group published a similar but much more comprehensive study.[2]

- That year, we also published, together with the center, the first phase I study on the safety of high-dose intravenous vitamin C in terminal cancer patients.[3]

In 2003, the NIH organized an international conference in Bethesda, Maryland, with the idea of generating a discussion among the world's experts on antioxidants and cancer in order to produce a research agenda. Among the speakers were two renowned scientists, Dr. Bruce Ames and Dr. David Golde. Dr. Ames' long and distinguished career included developing the Ames test, a system for testing the mutagenicity of compounds. Dr. Ames had produced many research publications on diverse scientific topics, including cancer and aging. Dr. Golde was the head of cancer research at Memorial Sloan-Kettering Cancer Center and had made important contributions in cancer research.

Michael was excited with the idea that we could discuss our disagreement with a concept presented in a paper by Dr. Golde's research team, which contributed to the notion that vitamin C could shield cancer cells from chemotherapy. They described for the first time how can-

cer cells absorb vitamin C by the same means as glucose (sugar) by uti-
lizing one of the glucose transporters (GLUT 1). However, at the end
of the article they made an unfortunate comment that vitamin C might
be a possible protector of cancer cells against the pro-oxidant effects of
chemotherapy. That comment, even though it was not actually part of
the study, contributed to the confusion over the role of vitamin C, and
antioxidants in general, in cancer. When we enrolled in the conference,
we were hoping to clarify this issue and demonstrate that the prepon-
derance of the evidence pointed to the contrary.

During one of the presentations, Michael wanted to comment on a
particular subject that we believed was important to elaborate, but we
realized that it was getting late and we had to get back to the hotel to
prepare for our poster session presenting one of our vitamin C studies.
We left the last presentation to find that there were no buses to take us
back, but we were told that a gentleman next to us had just called for a
taxi and he was going to our hotel. Michael looked at him and told me
it was Dr. Golde. So, I decided to ask him if we could share the taxi
with him and he agreed. After waiting for about ten minutes, the taxi
arrived. Dr. Golde then saw Dr. Ames in the crowd and invited him to
join us. Dr. Golde sat in the middle of the back seat, with Michael to
his left and me to his right. As soon as the taxi took off, Michael immediately took out our review paper on vitamin C and cancer. After
Michael pointed out that vitamin C can actually have pro-oxidant activity that can kill cancer cells, Dr. Golde put his hand to his head as he
pondered this information. His candid response was, "I did not know
this." At that moment, Dr. Bruce Ames turned his head toward us and
said, "You know, what these kids are saying is true. I was just talking to
the NIH expert on vitamin C, Dr. Mark Levine, about this." We invited Dr. Golde to be a co-author of our review paper on vitamin C.

OUR RESEARCH ON VITAMIN C AND CANCER

A 2005 publication from Dr. Levine's group at the NIH reported that
pharmacologic concentrations of ascorbic acid selectively kill cancer
cells.[4] It received worldwide attention because vitamin C is a relatively cheap, nontoxic nutrient with a history of being used as a therapeu-

tic tool against cancer. Nevertheless, this history has been full of controversy. The classical controversy was between Linus Pauling and Dr. Charles Moertel of the Mayo Clinic.[5] Varied results were published by the different camps, which initiated a seemingly neverending debate. The reality is that the studies were not done the same way—Dr. Moertel never replicated the Pauling experiments. Both studies used oral doses of vitamin C of about 10 grams, but Dr. Pauling also used intravenous administration of the vitamin. The oral doses given cannot reach plasma concentrations needed for vitamin C to achieve antineoplastic (cancer-fighting) activity.

Research on vitamin C and cancer generates continuously renewed interest, and there are several researchers working in this area. Dr. Levine's group has recently demonstrated that a regimen of daily pharmacologic ascorbate treatment significantly decreased growth rates of ovarian, pancreatic, and glioblastoma tumors in mice.[6]

A more recent controversy has ensued regarding vitamin C and conventional cancer treatment. There has been a concern that vitamin C might reduce the effectiveness of chemotherapy and radiation by reducing the potency of the free radicals generated by these therapies, which are necessary for killing the cancer cells. This misconception was due in part to the article published by Dr. Golde's group at Memorial Sloan-Kettering in 1999, in which they described how cancer cells acquire and concentrate vitamin C. They suggested that these intracellular concentrations of vitamin C may provide malignant cells with a "metabolic advantage."[7] This suggestion has been embraced by most practitioners without any questioning or further evaluation, although no data demonstrating this suggestion has ever been published.

In contrast, a vast body of literature challenging these suggestions has been published. The study by Dr. Levine validates our earlier 2002 results, in which we demonstrated in vitro antineoplastic activity by high concentrations of ascorbic acid (equivalent to intravenous gram-level doses in humans). The main mechanism of vitamin C killing cancer cells is, paradoxically, by acting as an oxidant, and not (in this case) as an antioxidant. In the oxidizing/reducing redox cycle in cancer cells, vitamin C cycles between ascorbate and dehydroascorbate. Vitamin C enters the cell through the glucose transporters as dehydroascorbic acid, and inside the cell it picks up an electron and is "reduced" or reconverted to ascorbic acid. In this process, hydrogen peroxide is produced within the cell. Cancer cells, unlike other cells, have low amounts of antioxidant enzymes, notably catalase. In a healthy cell, catalase would convert peroxide to oxygen and water. However, in a cancer cell, the peroxide quickly builds up to toxic levels and kills the cell. Cancer cells have a much higher uptake of vitamin C than other cells because vitamin C is structurally similar to glucose and can be actively transported by a high number of specialized glucose transporter pumps.

We have published an in vivo study with guinea pigs and a report on clinical cases also showing antineoplastic activity with high-dose vitamin C.[8] Moreover, we published the first clinical trial on the safety of high-dose intravenous vitamin C on terminal cancer patients.[9] We are very excited with these results and believe this may lead to a new era in research, education, and healing in an integrated manner and spur the development of effective, nontoxic cancer therapies. There is much more research to do, but the emerging light makes the future look brighter.

OUR CANCER TREATMENT PROGRAM

We believe that by changing the biochemical conditions that promote, develop, and sustain the malignant state, we can inhibit malignant cell proliferation, increase aerobic metabolism, and achieve re-differentiation (pressure the cancer cells to return to normal). The idea is to produce a body environment (your internal "terrain") that does not favor cancer cell growth and tumor development. An oxygen-rich, non-acidic, nutrient-dense environment is discouraging to cancer, as it will allow metabolic correction which may guide gene expression to provide the instruction for normal cell behavior. This is why our program (especially diet and supplementation) is so crucial in the management of this disease.

Our research indicates that vitamin C is just one of various substances that can have a selective effect in modulating cancer cell metabolism either toward re-differentiation or apoptosis (self-induced cell death). *Our goal in cancer treatment is to change the conditions that encourage abnormal growth.*

Food as Cancer Medicine

In medicine, we habitually underestimate the power of nutrition as part of the treatment of most chronic diseases, especially cancer. One of the reasons for this neglect is that nutrition typically has a gradual effect upon disease. Another reason is the lack of emphasis in this area in medical school curricula. Scientific supplementation and nutrition should be taught to medical students and be part of every oncology treatment. Nutrition is not only preventive—it also has a curative role. There are many conditions that develop precisely as a result of inadequate nutrition. The way you solve malnutrition is with better nutrition, including the use of relatively high supplemental doses. *That* is orthomolecular medicine. It is also common sense that seems to be all too uncommon.

Nutritional intervention can help:

- Minimize the secondary effects (toxics) of the oncology treatment.

- Reinforce the immune system to help treat the disease.

- Treat disease directly with appropriate management of macro- and micronutrients (orthomolecular medicine).

- Help with the recovery of the patient.

Biochemical Optimization

Dealing with cancer is very difficult for the patient and family members in so many ways. The emotional and psychological impact of having a potentially mortal condition, the social and financial implications, the physical distress of the disease itself, and the considerable adverse effects of conventional treatment make cancer one of the most feared and difficult diseases. So, if we are to help the cancer patient to cope with this disease in the most effective way, it is imperative that we use all the support and therapeutic tools that, to the best of our knowledge, will improve the quality of life of the patient and give him or her the best opportunity to improve in all the aspects of life. The most advanced cancer treatment facilities recognize the need for integration in order to attain the best possible results. A multidisciplinary approach is not just a collection of a wide array of professionals and specialists. It should also directly integrate the patient, family members, and caretakers in an active role at the very center of the effort. *Some integrated programs do this and yet will still refuse to use high oral and intravenous doses of vitamins and other nutrients.*

High doses are required. Low doses fail. Says Thomas Levy, M.D.: "The three most important considerations in effective vitamin C therapy are dose, dose, and dose. If you don't take enough, you won't get the desired effects." Again we say, low doses do not get clinical results. Any physician, nurse, or parent knows that a dose of antibiotics that is one-tenth, or one-hundredth, of the known effective dose will not work. Indeed, it is a cornerstone of medical science that dose affects outcome. This premise is universally accepted with pharmaceutical drug therapy, but not with vitamin therapy.

The focus of our discussion is on one of the most neglected areas in medicine: biochemical correction and optimization. Supplementation with vitamins, minerals, and other nutrients has been repeatedly demonstrated to be very useful in improving patient outcomes, and doing so safely and cost effectively. *The management of the cancer patient must also include orthomolecular (nutritional) medicine.* Doing so will improve the patient's response to conventional therapy, reduce adverse effects of conventional therapy, and improve quality of life.

There is pressing, urgent need. Chemotherapy drugs have come and gone; the five-year survival rate for cancer treated with chemo has remained virtually unchanged for decades. Unfortunately, just over 2 percent of all cancers respond to chemotherapy. Specifically, one scientific review concluded that "chemotherapy only makes a minor contribution to cancer survival. To justify the continued funding and availability of drugs used in cytotoxic chemotherapy, a rigorous evaluation of the cost-effectiveness and impact on quality of life is urgently required."[10]

Conventional medical treatments based on drugs and invasive procedures are most successful in treating acute illnesses and traumas.

Chronic diseases have been and remain a tremendous challenge. There is a large segment of the population looking for other ways to manage their disease. In order to improve the success of drugs in the management of chronic diseases, it is important to know, understand, and integrate other scientifically based strategies. To maintain health, the human body will need a relatively pure environment; nutritious, unprocessed, and well-balanced variety of foods; nutrient supplementation; exercise and rest; and stress management strategies.

The rational treatment of chronic disease should consider as a priority the correction of the underlying biochemical problem and metabolic deficiencies. Standard medical therapy often concentrates on neutralizing or opposing some aspects of the pathophysiologic processes and too often without correcting the underlying cause of the condition. The management of chronic disease must be aimed to optimization of functions. If radiation, surgery, and chemotherapy could do this, cancer would be virtually extinct.

Energy Factors

We believe that the altered energy metabolism of tumor cells can provide a target for a new, nontoxic, vitamin C–based chemotherapeutic approach. An increased glucose consumption rate has been observed in malignant cells. Otto Warburg postulated that the respiratory process of malignant cells was impaired and the transformation of normal cells to malignant ones was due to defects in the aerobic respiratory pathways. Interestingly, during cell differentiation (where cell energy level is high), there is an increased cellular production of oxidants that appear to provide one type of physiological stimulation for changes in gene expression, and may lead to a terminal differentiated state which overcomes malignancy.

The failure to maintain high ATP production (cell energy level) may be a consequence of oxidative inactivation of key enzymes, especially those related to the Krebs cycle and the electron transport system. A distorted mitochondrial function (transmembrane potential) may result. This aspect could be suggestive of an important mitochondrial involvement in the carcinogenic process.

Replenishing Factors

Other nutritional factors not directly related to energy that have demonstrated an inhibitory effect on cancer growth and tumor development include enzymes, omega-3 fatty acids, vitamin D, vitamin K, iodine, and probiotics.

CHAPTER 3

Food as Cancer Medicine

"Let food be your medicine
and the medicine be your food."
—HIPPOCRATES

The human body is certainly complex, but what it asks of us is very simple. An automobile is made up of about 14,000 parts and is also complex. Remarkably, all you do is turn the key and it starts. With your body, the ignition key is eating right. Good nutrition is good preventive maintenance, and more.

Unlike a car, your body is self-repairing. Even the medical profession admits that most illnesses go away when doctors do nothing at all. We respect physicians who are reluctant to interfere with the normal healing process. Believe it or not, during the nineteenth century there was a movement among some American doctors to see patients and give them pills containing no medicine. These doctors were very popular because fewer of their patients died! If good bedside manner and a placebo (a drugless sugar tablet) gets a cure, that's good. To do something harmless and be helpful is good medicine. Eating right is better still.

Good nutrition does not directly cure disease; the body does. You provide the raw materials and the inborn wisdom of your body makes the repairs. You provide the bricks and mortar and the mason builds the wall. Without supplies, the most skilled workman on Earth can build nothing. Without plenty of nutrients, the body can't either.

THE POWER OF NUTRITION

The field of medicine continues to underestimate the power of nutrition as a vital part of the treatment of chronic diseases. Scientific nutrition should be a part of every cancer treatment. Nutrition serves not only as a preventive measure but also has a curative role.

As stated previously, nutrition can help:

- Minimize secondary toxic effects of cancer treatments, such as burning, nausea, and hair loss
- Reinforce the immune system to help fight the disease
- Treat the disease directly with macro- and micronutrients
- Help speed recovery of the patient and improve his or her quality of life

Poor nutrition promotes the development of abnormal cell growth. Even if someone doubted this statement, there are few who would say that poor nutrition helps a cancer patient. By the time you are done reading this chapter, you will see that corrective nutrition (a diet high in fiber, complex carbohydrates, vitamins, minerals, and enzymes) helps restore optimal body biochemistry, allowing better physiological conditions that promote good health, and provides a hostile environment for cancer.

The big problem is that the prevailing eating habits of our society are high in empty calories (lots of fat, sugar, and refined products) and low in nutritionally dense foods. This deficient diet promotes a pre-pathological state of subclinical deficiencies that damages our metabolism and sets us up for cancer. This occurs by lowering our needed enzymatic activity due to lack of the necessary cofactor vitamins, minerals, and other nutrients. Proper enzymatic activity is important to promote the biochemical reactions that maintain the balance of the healthy state. A deficiency of nutrients can lead to a distortion of the function of the immune system and in the balance of hormones. Metabolic imbalance affects cellular communication, cellular receptors, inflammatory mediators, and growth factors in such a way that degeneration is promoted.

FOOD IS THE CORE OF YOUR HEALTH

"Man is a food-dependent creature," said Emanuel Cheraskin, M.D. "If you don't feed him, he will die. If you feed him improperly, part of him will die." There is no doubt about it: poor diet is a major cause of cancer development and a critical aspect to consider in patients dealing with this condition. Poor diet fails to supply the body with the nutrients needed to maintain healthy cells and tissues. A poor diet does not support a healthy immune system, and a weak immune system will be less able to defend against the onset of cancer. Also, a poor diet promotes obesity. Obesity severely disturbs the body's ability to regulate the complex interactions among diet, metabolism, physical activity, hormones, and growth factors.

The accumulation of excess body fat along with low levels of physical activity (and continued poor diet) promotes insulin resistance, a glucose-insulin disorder. This disorder is one step prior to diabetes and it affects the immune system, tissue healing, and glucose management—all important factors in the development of several conditions, including accelerated aging and cancer. The patient who has cancer must understand that a proper diet can improve his or her sense of well-being and support the immune system, while an improper diet can drain energy and promote tumor growth. We make the following dietary recommendations for cancer prevention and treatment:

- Consider oxygen to be part of the diet

- Drink pure water; it means better body function and performance

- Eat lots of colorful vegetables and fruits

- Whole grains (wholesome and unrefined) are the staple food of humans; limit your intake of refined carbohydrates

- Limit the intake of animal foods (milk, meat)

- Increase the intake of omega-3 fatty acids

- Avoid high-calorie, low-nutrient-content food (junk foods, candy, and soft drinks)

- Keep salt intake low, potassium intake high

OXYGEN IS PART OF THE DIET

The air we breathe is about 20 percent oxygen, but we are 100 percent dependent on it. Oxygen is so essential for life that the body will not survive more than a few minutes without it. It is not usually considered part of the diet by most people. But it is by us. We consider oxygen part of the diet so that you are careful about providing yourself enough quality and quantity of good fresh air. This is serious.

If you are a smoker, you are depleting your body of oxygen while breathing in a host of toxins, and you are paying dearly for this. Even if you do not smoke, it is worthwhile to consider the quality of the air you breathe. In order to do this adequately you should pay the most attention to where you sleep and where you work. Does the building provide a source of good, fresh air? "Sick building syndrome" refers to the ill effects caused by enclosed buildings with recirculating air of poor quality. What is the quality of the air in your home and neighborhood? Are there factories that produce contaminants? Intense automobile traffic? Are there other sources of air contamination?

If the conditions of the air in your work or home are not the best, consider creating a sanctuary were you can control the quality of the air at least in one room, most conveniently your bedroom or your office. You can do this by using air conditioning, air filters, and ionizers. If you decide to do this, take the time to compare the specifications, quality, and capacity of various different products available to make sure they can do the job. In addition, if you decide to create a sanctuary, you should take into consideration full-spectrum lighting and all the other elements that will help you create a pleasant environment, appropriate for relaxation and enjoyment.

Exercise is another way to oxygenate your body while you receive other benefits. Exercise is not negotiable; you either do it or you will be denied its benefits. And until the government taxes walking, exercise is also free! Exercise can and will allow the body to increase the amount of oxygen. Remember that oxygen is essential for cellular respiration in all aerobic organisms, including us. Oxygen is used in our cells' mitochondria to help generate the molecule of energy called adenosine triphosphate (ATP). Healthy cells like oxygen; cancer cells do not. There is your motivation.

PURE WATER FOR BETTER PERFORMANCE

Water is essential to life for hydration, metabolism, and detoxification. We have only two rules: drink lots of this fluid and make sure it is pure. How do you know you are drinking enough? Because you are visiting the restroom several times a day. Hydration is a key to metabolic correction and optimization at physiological, cellular-biochemical levels. Without proper hydration, circulation, kidney function, and gastrointestinal function will be impaired. You need water to form urine and water to form stool that is not constipating. At the cellular-biochemical level, reactions occur in a water environment, as your blood and body cells are all mostly composed of water. Humans are even conceived in a watery environment. Indeed, plenty of water is necessary for the adequate function of all the elimination routes—urine, feces, sweat, and even for proper hydration of the respiratory mucosa, which has to eliminate carbon dioxide through breathing. "Plenty" means eight or more glasses of water daily. You've probably heard that before, and it is true. It is also easy and cheap to do.

There is more to consider than quantity—water purity is also a concern. Public water supplies are usually treated with chlorine to keep the number of microbes under a certain level. This practice has eliminated from our lives the risks of waterborne diseases such as typhoid fever, cholera, and dysentery. However, the downside to this treatment is that when chlorine reacts with organic compounds in the water, it forms trihalomethanes (THMs), a group of compounds known to be carcinogenic. Scientific studies have linked THMs to increased risk of cancer. A small increase in the risk of bladder cancer, colorectal cancer, and leukemia has been reported in several studies.[1] Some investigations have found that chlorination byproducts may be linked to heart, lung, kidney, liver, and central nervous system damage.[2] Other research has linked THMs to reproductive problems and birth defects.[3] A study conducted in California found a miscarriage rate of 15.7 percent for women who drank five or more glasses of cold water containing more than 75 ppb (parts per billion) of THM, compared to a miscarriage rate of 9.5 percent for women with a low trihalomethane exposure.[4] Even taking a shower can be a problem if the water is too high in THMs. One study showed that a ten-minute shower produced more absorption of THMs through the skin than drinking five glasses of water.[5]

When looking at the evidence relating THMs and health risks, cancer should be a primary concern. For these reasons, the Environmental Protection Agency (EPA) has lowered the allowable total trihalomethanes in public water supplies to 80 ppb from the previous level of 100 ppb. In order to deal with this risk, get informed. You may not have to do anything if the THM level of your water is fine. If the level of THMs in your water supply is close to the upper limit, start looking for filter systems. You can find fairly inexpensive systems with carbon filters for the shower or water supply to your home that will dramatically reduce the levels of THMs.

How do you know the water you are drinking is pure? It might be a little tricky, and you have to do your homework. The first tool you have is free, and that is your sense of smell and taste. If water smells or tastes bad, it is usually a bad sign. Purifying systems, such as distillers or reverse osmosis filters, will do the trick. We are not concerned about water as a source of dietary minerals, because you will obtain them in your diet and supplements. However, good quality well water does contain valuable minerals, and some well water may have a smell (sulfur) that is not harmful. The guiding rule is to have your well water source checked.

Also, pay attention to the condition of the water when you are drinking bottled water. The quality of bottled water is supervised by the government to a certain extent; however, once the water leaves the production plant, storage conditions can have an impact on its quality, especially if the water is exposed, in plastic containers, to sun and/or heat for enough time. This also applies once you buy the bottle. Plastic bottles exposed to sun and heat can leach a substance known as phthalates. Although you will not have acute toxicity by occasionally drinking water with a modest amount of phthalates, chronic exposure may contribute to hormonal dysregulation. In addition, water in an opened bottle or other container that is left unrefrigerated for enough time may become a culture of harmful bacteria, as with unrefrigerated food. Chill it.

EAT A COLORFUL ASSORTMENT OF FRUITS AND VEGETABLES

Select foods of different colors (red, orange, yellow, green, blue, and purple) to give your body the full spectrum of cancer-fighting compounds as well as the nutrients needed for optimal function and protection against disease. Vegetables and fruits contain an all-natural, anti-carcinogenic cocktail, a vast number of substances (phytochemicals) known to protect against cancer.

Among the most important groups of phytochemicals are the pigments, which give foods their color. Carotenes are the red-yellow pigments found in vegetables such as carrots, peppers, yams, and tomatoes, as well as in fruits such as apricots, watermelons, and cherries. Carotenes are also found in green leafy vegetables such as spinach and in legumes, grains, and seeds. Over 600 carotenes exist in the nature including about 50 that the body can transform into vitamin A. Beta-carotene is the most active of the carotenes because more of it is converted to vitamin A, but other carotenes such as lutein and lycopene probably exert greater anti-cancer effects. The deeper the green color, the greater the concentration of carotenes. You cannot see the carotene in green vegetables because of the green coloration of chlorophyll, but it is there nonetheless.

Other important groups of plant pigments are the flavonoids. These compounds have anti-inflammatory, anti-allergenic, anti-viral, and anti-cancer properties. Good dietary sources of flavonoids include citrus fruits, berries, onions, parsley, legumes, green tea, and grape juice or wine.

Nearly half of all Americans fail to consume even a single serving of fruit in a day.[6] Only a minority actually achieve the "five daily" recommendations for fruits and vegetables. Virtually no one is eating enough of the fruits and vegetables that are most important in fighting cancer. The key dietary recommendation to reduce your risk of cancer is to consume liberal amounts of fruits and vegetables. Dr. Harold Foster did a study in which he looked at 200 people with cancer who had experienced a "spontaneous regression." He wanted to know if these lucky people did something different to help them achieve this so-called spontaneous regression and he found that about 87 percent of them had changed their diet to vegetarian.[7]

What is better, raw or cooked? Generally, we recommend eating fruits and most vegetables in their raw state. Many compounds with anti-cancer properties are found in much higher concentration in raw foods than in their cooked counterparts. As a rule, if it can be eaten raw, it probably should be eaten raw. It may not be wise to consume more than four servings per week of raw cabbage family vegetables (broccoli, cauliflower, and kale), as these foods in their raw state contain compounds that can interfere with thyroid hormone production (and may also produce too much gas). If you decide to cook your vegetables, steam them lightly or quickly stir fry in a small quantity of oil, in order to preserve as much of the healing phytochemicals as possible.

WHOLE GRAINS—THE STAPLE FOOD OF HUMANS

Whole grains are foods that contain all the essential parts and naturally occurring nutrients of the entire grain seed. Whole grains consist mainly of carbohydrates, although they also contain fibers, fatty acids, proteins, minerals, and vitamins. Carbohydrates are the main source of energy for the body and it is important to nourish the body with good quality carbohydrates that provide the needed energy without disturbing hormonal balance and energy metabolism.

When refined carbohydrates (commonly found in processed foods) are consumed, they often lack the nutrients needed for optimal metabolic activity. In addition, they increase blood glucose, which may increase tumor growth. In order to control the glucose boost from refined carbohydrates, more insulin is required; chronic insulin over-secretion leads to insulin resistance, which predisposes to diabetes.

Whole grains reduce risks of chronic diseases such as heart disease, stroke, diabetes, obesity, and cancer. A review of recent studies on whole grains and health demonstrate that whole grain intake is protective against cancer and other chronic diseases.[8]

Types of whole grains other than wheat include:

- Amaranth
- Barley
- Buckwheat
- Corn, including whole cornmeal and popcorn

- Millet
- Oats, including oatmeal
- Quinoa

- Rice (brown, wild, and colored)
- Rye
- Sorghum (milo)

Reduce Your Exposure to Contaminants

Chemical contaminants include pesticides, industrial chemicals, and disinfection byproducts. Pesticides are widely used in agriculture and have been linked to various types of cancer. High doses of some of these chemicals can cause cancer in animals. Fruits and vegetables sometimes contain very small amounts of pesticides. Some dangerous pesticides such as DDT (dichloro-diphenyl-trichloroethane) are now banned, but were widely used in the past. These chemicals break down very slowly, so they can accumulate in the environment, and in you. They eventually find their way up the food chain and are stored in our fatty tissues. Workers exposed to higher levels of pesticides in industry or farming may be at higher risk of certain cancers, particularly leukemias and lymphomas.

Some scientists think that these chemicals could suppress the immune system in people who are regularly exposed to them. So, you should keep in mind that even low levels of contaminants in food can have cumulative effects, especially in people who may be unknowingly exposed to other environmental toxins or who have their detoxification capabilities compromised due to the use of multiple medications or genetic susceptibility. Because of this, always wash fruits and vegetables before eating them; or, even better, eat organic produce. When you wash produce, a small amount of soap or dishwashing detergent added to the water will increase the removal of pesticides. Most pesticides are in an oil base that does not wash off in the rain or under plain water in your sink. Use soap and then, of course, rinse well.

Phthalates are a family of chemicals known as plasticizers because they are used to soften hard plastics to make them more flexible. Phthalates have been produced since the 1920s and used in everything from perfumes to pesticides and medical instruments to sex toys. They can be absorbed from food and water. Higher levels have been found in milk and cheese. They can also leach into a liquid that comes in contact with the plastic. Although the potential of acute toxicity is low, there is concern among the scientific community that low-level chronic exposure can cause endocrine gland disruption. For this reason, Europe has banned the use of some phthalates in toys.

Does everything cause cancer? No. But it is good sense to minimize your exposure to what may cause it.

LIMIT THE INTAKE OF ANIMAL FOODS

Many epidemiological studies from around the world have investigated the link between meat consumption and cancer risk, looking at total meat intake and also intakes of red meat (beef, lamb, pork, veal) and processed meats. Higher red meat intake may be a risk factor for hormone receptor–positive breast cancer among premenopausal women.[9] The majority of breast cancer is hormone receptor–positive (stimulated by higher levels of estrogen or progesterone circulating in the body) and the incidence of these tumors has been increasing in the United States.

Potentially carcinogenic compounds found in meats include N-nitroso compounds, heterocyclic amines, or polycyclic aromatic hydrocarbons. N-nitroso compounds (nitrosamines and nitrosamides) have been found to be potent carcinogens in animal studies, as have heterocyclic amines. These carcinogens and other substances in meats (nitrates, nitrites, saturated fat) may cause a host of problems in the body—increased DNA synthesis leading to cell proliferation, increased insulin-like growth factor, hormone imbalances, free radical damage—which may cause cancer.

Milk is a valued nutrient because it is one of the most complete foods, full of macro- and micronutrients. However, since this nutrient-dense food is intended to support the growth and development of infant animals, it is flooded with growth factors. It is not uncommon for adults to have gastrointestinal disturbances when they consume milk. In most people, this could be due to the development of lactose intolerance (lack of the enzyme that digests lactose, a type of milk sugar). This is a hint: the body is letting us know to stop eating this food. However, milk can be a problem for other reasons, including allergy to the protein casein and exposure to traces of antibiotics and hormones (rBST or BGH) used to increase milk production. All these are stressors to your body. The growth factors and hormones in milk can help in tumor cell proliferation. Therefore, milk (especially mother's milk) is better used by infants and better avoided in patients with cancer or at high risk.

INCREASE THE INTAKE OF OMEGA-3 FATTY ACIDS

Several clinical studies have clearly shown that the omega-3 polyunsaturated fatty acids eicosapentaenoic acid (EPA) and docosahexaenoic acid (DHA), the main components of fish oil, help inhibit the promotion and progression of cancer.[10] Their beneficial effect is particularly pronounced in hormone-dependent cancers, such as breast cancer and prostate cancer.

Saturated fatty acids contain only single carbon-carbon bonds. "Saturated" means they are full to capacity with hydrogen molecules. These are generally animal fats, but palm and coconut oils are also saturated. Unsaturated fatty acids have one or more carbon double bonds. Each of these could accept more hydrogen molecules, therefore they are considered "unsaturated." Most vegetable oils are unsaturated.

Monounsaturated means only one carbon double bond. An example is oleic acid, found in olives, peanuts, almonds, and avocados. Polyunsaturated fatty acids (PUFAs) have two or more carbon double bonds, such as typical vegetable oils. EPA is an omega-3 fatty acid, meaning that the first carbon double bond is located three carbons in from the far (omega) end of each molecule. Most vegetable oils that you eat are omega-6 fatty acids, such as linoleic acid. The two most common fish oil omega-3 fatty acids are EPA and DHA. A third, vegetarian omega-3 is called linolenic acid, found in linseed oil and more importantly in soybean oil and green leafy vegetables. Linolenic acid is slowly converted into both DHA and EPA in the body.

Omega-3 fatty acids are protective against cancer progression, while omega-6 PUFAs (such as arachidonic acid) may help promote the growth of cancer. The omega-3s are healthful in several ways:

- They produce an overall anti-inflammatory effect.[11]

- They positively affect gene expression in the control of cell growth, differentiation, apoptosis, angiogenesis, and metastasis.[12]

- They suppress excessive nitric oxide (NO) during inflammation and help prevent DNA damage.[13]

- They decrease the estrogen-stimulated growth of hormone-dependent cancer cells.[14]

- Fish oils improve insulin sensitivity and cell membrane fluidity to help prevent the spread of cancer.[15]

The Japanese have the world's longest life expectancy among all the Westernized cultures, perhaps because they eat a lot of fish and they also eat very little red meat. A way that the omega-3 fatty acids might work to prolong health is by getting into each cell membrane, making them more bendable, adaptable, and durable. Improved immune response is a benefit of fish oil consumption. Oily fish (trout, mackerel, salmon) are best and a little dab will do you: even an ounce or two every other day is helpful. Non-oily fish (cod, flounder, haddock) are also worth having, but you'd need to eat more of them, perhaps a regular serving (3 to 4 ounces) on alternate days. The *New England Journal of Medicine* reported that as little as 30 grams of even low-fat fish per day reduced the twenty-year death rate from coronary heart disease by 50 percent.[16] That is only about one ounce of fish daily, actually providing less than 300 mg of omega-3s each day. Alternatively, you could eat a lot of green leafy vegetables, and take an EPA supplement. Around 300–1,000 mg of EPA daily is frequently recommended.

AVOID HIGH-CALORIE, LOW-NUTRIENT-CONTENT FOODS

Sugar is a generic term used to identify simple carbohydrates, which include monosaccharides, such as fructose, glucose, and galactose, and disaccharides, such as maltose and sucrose (white table sugar). Sucrose is mainly considered a biologic fuel to generate energy within the cell. Complex carbohydrates are polysaccharides, which include starches and fiber. Polysaccharides take more time to digest; fiber usually is not digested.

When you eat any kind of carbohydrate, it is broken down into simple molecules by enzymes in the digestive tract so that it can be absorbed and reach the bloodstream. This process produces a gradual absorption of the blood glucose if you are eating a complex carbohydrate, especially if you are ingesting a wholesome product that contains a fair amount of fiber. This gradual process allows the body to secrete an amount of insulin that will facilitate the entrance of glucose from the blood into the cell, where it will be used to form energy. Part of the process of making energy molecules—adenosine triphosphate (ATP)—from glucose does not require oxygen. Those mechanisms are also present in cancer cells. However, there are other mechanisms of making ATP that require oxygen that are unavailable to the cancer cell. Therefore, in terms of energy, you can say that normal cells are like hybrid automobiles—they are more fuel efficient because they have two systems of generating energy: oxygen-dependent and also anaerobic (without oxygen).

Carbohydrates are one of the macronutrients essential to life along

The Trouble with Sugar

Excessive intake of sugar can lead to a host of significant health problems. High levels of sugar can:

- Suppress immune function.

- Lead to deficiencies of chromium, copper, calcium, and magnesium.

- Increase adrenaline levels, a factor in hyperactivity and anxiety.

- Elevate levels of cholesterol and triglycerides.

- Suppress enzyme function in the body.

- Cause hormone imbalances.

- Increase free radical formation and oxidative damage.

- Contribute to vision problems, gastrointestinal difficulties (indigestion, increased risk of Crohn's disease, and ulcerative colitis), cardiovascular disease and hypertension, periodontal disease, obesity, osteoporosis, autoimmune diseases (arthritis and multiple sclerosis), headaches, depression, yeast infections, and Alzheimer's disease.

And if you have one of these conditions, sugar is sure to make it worse.

with proteins and fats. You cannot even think straight when blood sugar goes down because the brain needs glucose for proper functioning. There is no question about the importance of carbohydrates in the diet; *the question is about the quality and quantity of carbohydrates.*

When people consume more sugar than necessary, and the ingestion is in the more refined forms, blood glucose will rise much faster, which will require more insulin. Exposure to substantial amounts of refined sugar beyond the body's needs will lead to insulin resistance, overweight, and even diabetes. In addition, you will be providing the best nutrition to cancer cells. Sugar has been connected with the development of cancers of the breast, ovaries, prostate, rectum, pancreas, gallbladder, and stomach. The concept that sugar feeds cancer is almost totally overlooked as part of most conventional comprehensive cancer treatment plans. Not by us. Sugar is not your friend.

Unfortunately, cancer patients are rarely offered any significant nutritional therapy or advice. Controlling one's intake of cancer's preferred fuel, glucose, could prove beneficial in slowing the cancer's

The Importance of the Glycemic Index

The glycemic index is a system used to rate the speed at which a given food increases blood glucose levels. The faster the rise, the higher the glycemic index. The slower the increase in blood sugar, the lower the glycemic index. Generally, slower sugar absorption into the bloodstream means better utilization by tissues. If a person consistently eats to provoke rapid blood sugar increases, this constitutes a severe bodily stress. Unabated, it can alter body hormonal balance and lead to diabetes, obesity, yeast overgrowth, and cardiovascular problems.

Given the role of sugar as a main fuel in the cancer cell, it is important to keep sugars limited to fulfill basic body needs but not taken in excess, which can feed the rapidly reproducing cancer cells. Therefore, the diet should contain lots of vegetables and the least possible sugars. For those moments when we crave a sweet taste, a modest amount of intensely colored, nutrient-rich fruits are the best bet. This is not just health-nut sugar bashing. Rats fed a high-sugar diet develop more cases of breast cancer.[17]

growth. This would give the immune system a better chance to fight the cancer's growth and allow other medical modalities to be more effective in reducing tumor size. Diet, supplements, and exercise to normalize sugar should be part of any cancer treatment program.

You recall that it was 1931 Nobel Prize winner Otto Warburg, Ph.D., who postulated that the energy production in cancer cells is abnormal compared to healthy cells. They tend to emphasize anaerobic (without oxygen) metabolism, in which glucose is consumed by cancer cells and large amounts of lactic acid results as a waste product. This produces a more acidic pH in cancer tissues and greater physical fatigue. This lactic acid can be reconverted to glucose, but the metabolic energy expended is enormous. This is why cancer is a "wasting" disease—the person with cancer becomes continually more tired and undernourished, leading to cachexia.

That's why it is so important that any approach to cancer encompass regulating blood sugar through eating a healthful, low-sugar diet, taking nutritional supplements, and exercising to help normalize blood sugar. The goal is to control blood sugar in order to starve cancer cells of their favorite fuel and to help improve the immune system's ability to fight the cancer.

In a clinical study with ten healthy volunteers, fasting blood glucose and phagocytic index of neutrophils were determined. The phagocytic index measures the capacity of immune cells to neutralize invaders such as cancer. When given 100 grams of carbohydrates from glucose, sucrose, honey, and orange juice, all saw a significantly decreased capacity of neutrophils. Starch did not have this effect.[18]

An animal study using mice with human breast cancer showed that tumors are sensitive to blood sugar levels. An aggressive strain of breast cancer was injected into sixty-eight mice and they were then fed diets to induce either high, normal, or low blood sugar. A dose-dependent response was found: the lower the blood sugar, the greater the survival rate.[19] An epidemiological study performed in twenty-one countries, including Europe, North America, and Japan, found that sugar intake was a strong risk factor that contributes to higher breast cancer rates, especially in older women.[20]

KEEP SALT INTAKE LOW, POTASSIUM INTAKE HIGH

A high-sodium, low-potassium diet can cause high blood pressure and may also increase cancer risk. *The optimal dietary potassium-to-sodium ratio should be 5:1.* This is about ten times more potassium than the average intake. Bananas and oranges are high in potassium. In fact, most fruits, vegetables, and plant foods (indeed, most unprocessed whole foods) are fair to very good sources of potassium. The most common food additive is salt, and salt means sodium.

Tips for eating less salt:

- Reduce the salt you use gradually as this will help you get used to the change in flavor.

- Look for low-salt, no added salt, and salt-reduced products.

- To add flavor to meals, use garlic, onion, chili powder, lemon juice, vinegar, pepper, herbs, curry paste, spices, or a strongly flavored oil, such as sesame, mustard seed, or extra-virgin olive oil.

- Buy unsalted nuts.

- If you must use salt, use only small amounts of very salty ingredients (such as olives or anchovies) in cooking, and chop them finely to ensure their flavor is mixed well throughout the dish.

THE IMPORTANCE OF DETOXIFICATION

Since a long-term buildup of waste products may promote cancer, we think a "detox diet" is wise. It helps your body's organs work at an optimal level, without obstruction. A detoxification program usually involves lots of fiber and lots of water. Abundant dietary fiber helps your colon to much more easily remove waste. This, in turn, gives you relief and more energy. If you do not believe this, try it and see. Water has an overall beneficial effect on how well your body functions. Instead of letting waste build up and cause problems, the detox diet rids your body of waste and allows your entire gastrointestinal tract to work optimally once again, from one end to the other.

Successful therapies against cancer will result in the death of tumor cells. These dead tumor cells and their contents are highly toxic and must be removed by the body. It is possible that toxicity from the death of many tumor cells, as can happen in chemotherapy or other anti-cancer therapies, can harm or even kill a cancer patient if the body is not detoxified.

If a cancer patient is getting headaches, nausea, chills, fever, and other symptoms, which often relate to the inability to detoxify efficiently, then the following steps may help.

1. Consider supplementing with coenzyme Q_{10} (coQ_{10}), which can increase the efficiency of the heart, boost immune function, increase energy in the body, and provide many more benefits. The different abilities of coQ_{10} can enhance detoxification. For example, coQ_{10} can help increase blood volume. Red blood cells carry away detoxified substances, and increasing the volume of blood can enhance the rapid elimination of toxins.

2. Consider supplementing with olive leaf extract. There are two systems of immune function, called the T helper 1 and T helper 2 systems. The T helper 1 system deals with viruses, bacteria, cancer cells, and other organisms. If a person is susceptible to viral infection, bacterial infection, and cancer cells, this may be an indicator of a weak T helper 1 system. Olive leaf has been shown to be antiviral and antibacterial. Strengthening the T helper 1 system can help fight against cancer cells.

3. Consider supplementing with trimethylglycine (TMG), which helps promote methylation. Methylation is an important chemical process in the body that involves proper metabolism of methionine and cysteine, two amino acids needed for detoxification.

4. Consider supplementing with ion-exchange whey protein powder. Whey has been shown in some studies to boost immune function.[22] It also supplies 98 percent of the essential amino acids that the body needs. Amino acids are a primary method to detoxify the body, and whey can supply the necessary amounts.

5. Consider supplementing with silymarin from milk thistle (*Silybum*

The Gerson Cancer Therapy

The Gerson therapy is an intensive nutritional treatment of cancer and other life-threatening diseases, which has produced remarkable results that many would consider to have been impossible to obtain. Thanks to the work of Max Gerson, M.D., and his daughter, Charlotte Gerson, this knowledge is readily available for all who need it.

Dr. Gerson (1881–1959) cured cancer with a strict fat-free, salt-free, low-protein, essentially vegetarian dietary regimen, based on great quantities of fresh vegetable juice, supplements, and systemic detoxification. As Charlotte Gerson explains in her book, *The Gerson Therapy:* "Dr. Gerson found that the underlying problems of all cancer patients are toxicity and deficiency. . . . He found that one of the important features of his therapy had to be the hourly administration of fresh vegetable juices. These supply ample nutrients, as well as fluids to help flush out the kidneys. When the high levels of nutrients re-enter tissues, toxins accumulated over many years are forced into the bloodstream. The toxins are then filtered out by the liver."

Dr. Gerson found that he could provide help to the liver overwhelmed by these toxins using the caffeine in coffee absorbed from the colon, which carries the caffeine to the portal system and then to the liver. The caffeine stimulates the liver/bile ducts to open, releasing the poisons into the intestinal tract for excretion.

The Gerson Therapy consists of treatment specifics, cautions, recipes, case histories, and references. The book contains explicit instructions for the administration of the crucial liver-detoxifying coffee enemas. The use of castor oil, a thorough listing of which foods to eat (and not eat), how to juice, psychological aspects of therapy, and generally favorable mentions of megadose vitamin C supplementation are also presented. Dosage and rationale for the supplements Dr. Gerson prescribed—potassium, iodine, digestive enzymes, niacin, thyroid and liver extracts (by prescription), and vitamin B_{12} injections—are all covered.

The Gerson therapy is not specifically a cancer treatment. Dr. Gerson saw it as a metabolic treatment, one that cleanses the human organism while strengthening the body's ability to heal itself. Not surprisingly, therefore, the Gerson therapy is effective against a wide variety of diseases and for prevention as well.[21]

marianum). Silymarin helps improve liver function, and the liver is your body's main organ of detoxification.

6. Consider drinking 8–12 glasses of distilled water. Water is a primary method of detoxification in the body. Water also helps support kidney function by diluting urine. The proper amount of water decreases stress on the kidneys. Your urine should be clear to indicate you are getting the right amount of water.

7. Multiple bowel movements daily can help clear some of the toxic load your body must handle each day. This can decrease stress and help free energy to detoxify. Using vitamin C, vitamin B5 (pantothenic acid), and magnesium supplements can help you have multiple bowel movements each day. Take orthomolecular doses for best results: vitamin C to bowel tolerance, vitamin B5 (1 gram daily, in divided doses), and magnesium (500–1,000 mg daily, in divided doses). Vitamin C can accomplish bowel movements by itself, but a combination may make the stools proper in size and not too soft.

8. Consider supplementing with B-complex vitamins, 2–3 times a day. The B-complex is vital in detoxification of the cells.[23]

9. Consider supplementing with lycopene, a natural pigment synthesized by plants and microorganisms that has powerful antioxidant properties. A member of the carotenoid family, lycopene has been found to offer protection from both cancer and heart disease. In men with prostate cancer, lycopene supplementation has been found to lower levels of prostate-specific antigen (PSA), a widely used marker of prostate cancer progression and response to treatment.[24] Epidemiological studies have suggested that lycopene has a protective effect against breast cancer. Low levels of lycopene in the diet and in blood have been correlated with an increased risk of breast cancer.[25]

10. Consider supplementing with antioxidants, which help support detoxification, in optimal doses. Vitamins C and E, glutathione, alpha-lipoic acid, selenium, and pycnogenol are major antioxidants. Pycnogenol seems to help the other primary antioxidants work better.

11. Consider using bicarbonate whenever you get reactions or symptoms. Bicarbonate helps to regulate acid balance in the body. Antioxidants and other nutrients work better when there is proper acid-alkaline balance. Use one-eighth to one-quarter teaspoon of baking soda in distilled water.

GENERAL DIETARY GUIDELINES

- Fresh air and exercise are no-brainers for improved well-being. Get out in the country whenever you possibly can, breathe deep, and fill your lungs with oxygen the natural way.

- Drink an abundance of pure water and a limited amount of natural juices without added sugar. No sodas. No artificial sweeteners either.

- Eat *at least* two portions of fruit daily, but only on an empty stomach, first thing in the morning. More is better.

- Eat *at least* five, and preferably far more, servings of vegetables per day, especially greens, reds, purples, and yellows.

- Eat pulses (beans and lentils) at least three times per week. More is better.

- Only eat whole grains like whole oats, brown rice, barley, or millet. Sprouted grains are highly recommended.

- Avoid all sugar, especially glucose. Again we say, no soft drinks.

- Eat fresh nuts and seeds (especially pumpkin, sunflower, and linseeds). Chew them very well.

- Use fresh oils, especially olive oil or walnut oil. Recommended fats include extra-virgin, cold-pressed, organic olive oil, avocado oil, and extra-virgin, cold-pressed, organic coconut oil. No margarine or other partially hydrogenated oils (they contain unhealthy trans-fatty acids); no corn oil. Smell them to be sure the oils are fresh.

- Radically restrict your use of salt. Cut out as many processed, prepared, canned, and packaged foods as you possibly can. Remember: salt is the number one processed food additive. Therefore, avoid potato chips, peanuts, sausages, bacon, soy sauce and other condi-

ments, and especially Chinese food made with monosodium gluta-
mate (MSG).

- Limit your consumption of red meat and focus instead on consum-
  ing oily fish (such as salmon or trout). Organically farmed meats and
  fish have fewer added drugs or pesticides.

- Avoid milk and other dairy foods, especially if your cancer is hor-
  monally driven (breast, prostate, colon, etc.). Yogurt is okay.

- Drink 3–4 cups of green tea per day, and a glass or two of red wine
  per week. Grape juice is good, too.

- Take a daily probiotic supplement, ideally containing several different strains of friendly bacteria.

- Do not fry foods at high temperatures. Grill or, better yet, steam
  where possible. Eat at least one raw meal per day.

- Graze. Eat five to six small meals per day, rather than one or two big
  ones.

CHAPTER 4

Biochemical Optimization for Cancer Patients

"All truth passes through three stages:
First, it is ridiculed;
second, it is violently opposed; and
third, it is accepted as being self evident."
—ARTHUR SCHOPENHAUER (1788–1860)

When dealing with cancer or any chronic disease, there is no sub-stitute for proper eating. Eating healthy is critical for improving your health at any age. While staying active is also important, eating the wrong kind or wrong quantity of food will compromise your health. For example, if you have joint pain due to osteoarthritis, there is going to be inflammation and some level of cartilage degeneration. Foods that contain considerable amounts of arachidonic acid, such as dairy and eggs, will promote inflammation, thus increasing pain and promoting mobility problems.

Dietary changes tend to work slowly and do not always achieve the desired level of improvement. Supplementation is the next step to bringing further benefits. In some cases, dietary supplements can achieve benefits that cannot be obtained by other means, even by med-ications. For example, the only way to halt cartilage deterioration in patients with arthritis (as demonstrated by several prospective, ran-domized trials) is using a supplement called glucosamine sulfate.[1]

In the case of cancer, we have already discussed the negative effects of simple sugars, milk, and other refined products. In order to get the best results, it is important to adjust the diet to produce major changes that will improve the body's biochemical-functional environment. In some patients, diet alone may achieve the desired results. However, given the genetic diversity and the complex interactions with other internal and external factors that influence disease, most people will require additional nutritional fine-tuning that can be achieved through scientific dietary supplementation (orthomolecular therapy).

The use of supplements is a concept that originated several decades ago. Dr. Roger Williams (1893–1988) was a pioneer in biochemistry, nutrition, and biochemical individuality who discovered the vitamin pantothenic acid. When he was in his eighties, after a life of outstanding achievements, Dr. Williams wrote *The Wonderful World Within You: Your Inner Nutritional Environment*, a book that increased the awareness of the potential of nutrients in improving health.[2] But even now, twenty years after his death, much of his late work is still not appreciated.

Dr. Williams established the concept that to sustain life, humans share the same general biochemical metabolic pathways, but these pathways are not all equally efficient. These apparently small differences explain individual susceptibilities to certain diseases or exceptional resistance in certain people. The implication is that if we provide the system with the most essential elements needed for biochemical reactions to take place, the end product will form in the amount sufficient to meet the demand for a specific body function.

Another pioneer who contributed to promoting specific nutrients in treating health problems was Dr. Linus C. Pauling, a two-time Nobel Prize laureate. He coined the term *orthomolecular medicine* in 1968, by which he meant giving the body optimal amounts of natural substances in order to treat disease. Genes affect not only the physical appearance of people, but also their internal biochemistry. Diseases such as atherosclerosis, cancer, and depression are due to biochemical imbalances.

Biochemical optimization is a great tool to achieve optimal health when you use it as part of an integrated plan that combines diet, exercise, stress management, and spirituality. Understanding biochemical individuality is key to promoting biochemical optimization, which greatly facilitates the improvement of health.

THE ROLE OF METABOLISM

Everybody knows that living organisms need nutrients to sustain life and reproduce. Nutrients are compounds in food that the organisms need to live and grow. If you think about it, the oxygen in the air we breathe and the water we drink are usually not considered as nutrients, but certainly fit the definition because without them we would not last long. On the other hand, refined carbohydrates and sugars, which are widely consumed in our society, should not even be considered nutrients—on the contrary, they are macronutrients without micronutrients. We like to call these "anti-nutrients" to emphasize the fact that these edible substances will provide empty calories at the cost of wasting micronutrient reserves used up in the process of absorption and assimilation. In other words, anti-nutrients will provide empty calories with a net loss of micronutrients. Since these products are so widely consumed, it is no wonder that depletion of micronutrients may be causing a plethora of chronic health problems. Understanding the role of nutrients in metabolism is important in order to use this knowledge to control disease and increase wellness by optimizing metabolism.

Metabolism refers to chemical reactions that help the body grow, reproduce, repair injuries, and rebuild. Anabolism is the use of energy to build molecules, while catabolism is the breaking down of large molecules. Metabolic reactions involve pathways in which chemicals are transformed by enzymes, special proteins that catalyze chemical reactions and couple energy-consuming ones to more efficient ones. It's like putting lubricant on a mechanism to allow easier functioning, thus requiring less energy.

Most metabolic reactions involve transferring functional groups. For example, in a methyl group, a carbon atom is surrounded with hydrogen. When a methyl group is added to a particular molecule, it changes its activity. DNA methylation is of particular interest because evidence suggests that it has important therapeutic applications in cancer. This allows cells to use metabolic intermediates—cofactors or coenzymes—to move functional groups between reactions. The cofactors are continuously being used and recycled for additional reactions.

These coenzymes need vitamins and minerals as part of their structure in order to function. Vitamins and minerals act as catalysts in metabolism. There are seventeen required minerals (essential minerals) to support cell structure and function in human biochemical processes. There are two kinds of minerals: macrominerals and trace minerals. The macromineral group includes calcium, phosphorus, magnesium, sodium, potassium, chloride, and sulfur. The trace minerals include iodine, iron, copper, selenium, zinc, and others. Most nutritionists believe that the requirements for minerals are met simply with a conventional balanced diet. However, this ignores biochemical individuality and failure to understand this may not allow you to reach metabolic optimization.

- Deficiencies of certain nutrients—vitamins B_{12}, B_6, C, and E, folic acid, iron, and zinc—can damage DNA (deoxyribonucleic acid) in a similar way to radiation, by causing DNA breaks and/or free radical damage. Half of the population may be deficient in at least one of these micronutrients.

- As many as fifty genetic diseases are due to a poor link between enzymes and their cofactors or coenzymes. High-dose B vitamins can increase levels of these coenzymes.

- Free radical damage to mitochondria is a major factor in aging, but it can be helped by increasing intake of mitochondrial metabolites, such as coenzyme Q_{10}, carnitine, and lipoic acid, at high levels. Many common micronutrient deficiencies can accelerate deterioration of mitochondrial function, which seems to be a major contributor to cancer and aging.[3]

The optimum intake of micronutrients for each person varies according to age and genetic constitution, diseases, and exposure to stress or toxins. An optimum intake of micronutrients could tune up metabolism and give a marked increase in health.[4]

METABOLIC OPTIMIZATION

Every part of your body's physiology and function needs to be addressed in order for you to reach peak efficiency. Each part of the metabolic processes in the body are like links in a chain, and your strength can be compromised by one weak link. Metabolic optimization can help you recover faster and have more energy, thereby reducing the number of illnesses.[5]

Few people in the industrialized world have nutrient deficiency diseases (pellagra, rickets, scurvy, beriberi), but that doesn't mean that everyone is getting enough vitamins from their diet. In fact, a significant portion of the American population does not get the Recommended Dietary Allowance (RDA)—the minimal amount needed for health—of many critical nutrients. These so-called subclinical deficiencies can lead to serious health problems. Supplementation with specific nutrients has been estimated to be cost effective in preventing disease.[6]

Oral nutritional supplementation of acutely ill, hospitalized, older patients led to a statistically significant benefit in quality of life.[7] Diet by itself may not provide sufficient micronutrients to prevent deficiencies—that is, it may not even meet the RDA standards.[8] Researchers found that:

- 100 percent of diets were deficient in iodine

- 95 percent of diets were deficient in vitamin D

- 80 percent of diets were deficient in zinc

- 65 percent of diets were deficient in vitamin E

- 50 percent of diets were deficient in calcium

A large proportion of older adults do not consume sufficient amounts of many nutrients from foods alone.[9] Studies examining nutrient intakes in elderly who receive home-delivered meals and in other community-dwelling elderly have shown inadequate intakes of calcium, magnesium, protein, thiamine (vitamin B_1), vitamin C, and zinc. The associated cardiac disease risk implications of hypomagnesemia, and the increased risk of hip fracture with low calcium and vitamin D intake, make these findings particularly worrisome.[10] Supplements compensate to some extent, but only an estimated half of this population uses them daily.[11]

When even one micronutrient component falls short, it can affect a number of metabolic processes in the body and lead to illness. For example, mitochondrial damage may result in cancer, as well as cognitive dysfunction (from neuron decay), accelerated aging, and Alzheimer's disease. Those with genetic diseases due to defective enzymes may benefit from high doses of the B vitamin associated with the linked coenzyme, which can restore some of the enzymatic activity.

Cell Energy Production

Adenosine triphosphate (ATP) is the form of energy produced and stored in the cells' mitochondria, the energy currency for all the body's reactions. ATP from carbohydrates is produced in three steps.

- The initial step is called glycolysis, which does not require oxygen (anaerobic) and produces a small net gain of energy molecules. Rapidly growing malignant cells have glycolytic rates that are up to 200 times higher than normal tissues. Cancer may primarily be caused by a dysfunction in mitochondrial metabolism, which disrupts normal gene expression leading to uncontrolled growth of cells.[12]

- The Krebs cycle is a series of enzymatic energy-producing reactions that use oxygen for cellular respiration. It produces more energy per glucose molecule and occurs within the mitochondria. The Krebs cycle creates a form of energy that is transferable to every system in the body, but it is limited by the availability of reactants, minerals, and enzymes.

- The third energy-producing process, called oxidative phosphorylation, is a highly efficient way of releasing energy that moves electrons from electron donors to acceptors, such as oxygen (reduction/oxidation or redox reactions).

DNA Methylation

In DNA methylation, a methyl group is added to a carbon molecule in the DNA bases. This results from the activity of DNA methyltransferase enzymes. Alterations in methylation are commonly considered changes in gene expression, or epigenetic changes, which can affect the structure of DNA. The importance of this is that DNA methylation appears to be altered in cancer. The genes in tumor cells seem to be less methylated than normal cells. So, mechanisms involved in methylation can be targeted for potential cancer therapies, including tumor suppressors, angiogenesis inhibitors, and repair enzymes. Down-regulation of parts of DNA methylation, perhaps through drug therapies, could also inhibit cancer growth.[13]

Using anti-cancer agents to increase methylation of tumor suppressor genes holds promise, as do methylation inhibitors. Cancer hypermethylation and hypomethylation target tumor growth at different stages, and this has clear implications regarding potential anti-cancer therapies.[14]

In summary, the concept of metabolic optimization goes beyond the correction of underlying biochemical disturbances or deficiencies. These deficiencies can affect cell energy production, cell signaling to the nucleus, and ultimately gene expression. Metabolic optimization intends to improve such processes to a point that the biochemical correction is swift, while at the same time providing the physiological benefits of increased energy level, enhanced immunity, and an overall sense of well-being.

METABOLIC SUPPLEMENTATION FOR THE CANCER PATIENT

The scientific combination of proper nutrition and supplementation is mandatory in an integrative oncology treatment protocol for every cancer patient. So, in addition to the dietary recommendations in the last chapter, the following dietary supplements are recommended.

- A high potency multivitamin/mineral supplement. This is the basic supplement that should be taken by all people with a degenerative disease. It should provide all the recognized nutrients in high doses, such as the B-complex vitamins and minerals like zinc and magnesium needed as cofactors to improve the biochemical milieu. This is important for facilitating the flow of reactions leading to the formation of energy molecules. The B complex is also important in the reduction of homocysteine and other inflammatory molecules, in addition to controlling DNA methylation. A good formula should contain quality ingredients such as organic selenium, vitamin E as mixed tocopherols with tocotrienols, and mixed carotenoids. We clarify this because there are a lot of brands that use the less expensive forms of nutrients, which are less absorbed and/or have reduced biological activity. Take once a day with food.

- Vitamin C. Take 3,000–5,000 mg minimum daily in divided doses. There is a wide variety of forms of vitamin C. Some, such as the mineral ascorbates, may be more tolerable and are non-acidic. They are also more expensive than regular ascorbic acid. There is more information on vitamin C and cancer below.

- Coenzyme Q_{10}. Take the ubiquinol form of coQ_{10}; 100–300 mg daily.

- R-Lipoic acid. Take 300 mg once or twice a day.

- Acetyl-L-carnitine. Take 500 mg once or twice a day.

- Omega-3 fish oil. Take 500 mg of eicosapentaenoic acid (EPA) and 700 mg of docosahexaenoic acid (DHA) three times a day, with meals.

- Iodine. Take 25 mg once daily.

- High-potency digestive enzymes. Your food is only as good as its digestion. To help your body do the job better, take 2–4 tablets, two hours before or after a meal.

- Probiotics. A probiotic is the opposite of an antibiotic. A probiotic promotes beneficial bacterial growth. Use formulas with multiple strains of friendly bacteria, along with fructooligosaccharides (FOS), two hours before or after a meal. A target dose of 2–4 billion viable organisms is usually achieved with several tablets or capsules.

- Quercetin. Quercetin is a flavonoid, one of the plant pigments that give color to fruits and vegetables. This compound is found in medicinal plants, including *Ginkgo biloba* and St. John's wort. It is an antioxidant and has been found to have antihistaminic and anti-inflammatory properties. Laboratory and epidemiological studies suggest that quercetin also has cancer-preventing properties. Quercetin and other flavonoids have shown in animal and test tube studies to inhibit the growth of different types of cancer cells, including breast,[15] leukemia,[16] colon,[17] ovary,[18] gastric,[19] and non-small-cell lung cancer.[20] Take 200–400 mg daily.

- Vitamin D. Take 5,000 IU daily.

- Selenium. Selenium is a trace mineral that is essential for health but required only in small amounts. Selenium is incorporated into proteins to make selenoproteins, which are important antioxidant enzymes. Studies show that death from cancer, including lung, colorectal, and prostate cancers, is lower among those with higher blood levels or intake of selenium.[21] Take 200–400 mcg daily.

- Green tea. Take as desired. There is more information on green tea and cancer below.

Keep in mind that while these core nutrients may be beneficial for most patients, by virtue of biochemical individuality there might be a need for other specific nutrients or for higher amounts. Lacking a specific nutrient will cause biochemical and physiological derangements, which can only be properly treated by giving the correct amount of that specific nutrient. Dietary supplementation is often used successfully by many people, either by self-medication or by professional recommendation. One of the most important indications of success is achieving the desired clinical outcome. However, in the case of conditions such as cancer, you need expert help from competent professionals to monitor the state of your condition. Even when achieving the desired clinical outcome, you might not achieve the biochemical optimization ultimately needed for true healing. The best professional judgment should be based on a rational application of the current scientific and medical evidence, along with individual patient information. In order to follow the orthomolecular therapy that will work the best, laboratory testing is needed.

OTHER BENEFICIAL SUPPLEMENTS

The following is a list of other important nutrients that have a role in cancer prevention and treatment.

Chlorophyll

Chlorophyll is a green pigment found in most plants. It is vital for photosynthesis, the process that allows plants to obtain energy from light and convert nutrients from the soil into the macronutrients. The key function of this molecule is a redox reaction in which the chlorophyll donates an electron into molecular intermediates that produce energy molecules. Chlorophyll is structurally similar to heme, the molecule (of hemoglobin) that carries oxygen in the blood, but instead of having iron in its center, it has magnesium. Several studies have documented the anti-cancer activity of chlorophyll by more than one mechanism. Researchers indicate that chlorophyll acts as an interceptor molecule in order to block the absorption of aflatoxins (known carcinogens) and other cancer-causing constituents in the diet.[22] This molecular trapping reduces the body's exposure to the carcinogen.[23] Evidence suggests that individual chlorophyll derivatives have cytotoxic activities against tumor cells.[24]

Vitamin K

Recent research has demonstrated the anti-cancer action of vitamin K, which may act by modulating various transcription factors, leading to cell cycle arrest and cell death.[25] Findings also suggest that vitamin K_3 induces the arrest of a cell cycle (at the G2/M phase) and thus it may be useful for enhancing drugs that work in that phase.[26]

Carotenoids

Various natural carotenoids (organic plant pigments), besides beta-carotene, have been proven to have anticarcinogenic activity, and some of them showed more potent activity than beta-carotene.[27] Research indicates that the anticarcinogenic effects are related to a significant inhibition in the synthesis of nucleic acids in malignant human cell lines and disruption in DNA–protein interactions.[28] The antiproliferative activity of some retinoids may be due to their ability to modify gene expression.[29]

Curcumin

Cancer-related activities of curcumin, from the Indian spice turmeric, are linked to its known antioxidant and pro-oxidant properties. Its action has a potential to destroy a tumor directly by apoptosis (programmed cell death).[30] Curcuminoids can interfere with several cell-signaling pathways that may be useful in fighting cancer growth.[31] The anti-cancer activity of curcumin is attributable to a transcription factor that affects cell survival and angiogenesis (growth of blood vessels) in tumors.[32]

Garlic

Recent studies have shown that certain naturally occurring sulfur-containing compounds found in garlic can suppress proliferation of cancer cells. They do this by interfering in cell cycle progression (induction of G2/M phase)[33] and by interfering with cell division of the cancer cells.[34]

Green Tea

Camellia sinensis or green tea has been widely used for centuries in Asia. Green tea promotes the burning of fat by causing carbohydrates to be released slowly. This prevents sharp increases in blood insulin levels. Polyphenols in tea inhibit the production of enzymes that break down sugar. This reduces both glucose and insulin levels, and it can be helpful to people predisposed to diabetes and heart disease, or who are overweight.[35] Traditional medical systems claim that this plant has beneficial effects in the management of disease conditions, including asthma, angina pectoris, peripheral vascular disease, and coronary artery disease.

The anticarcinogenic effects of tea relate specifically to the catechins. Catechins (also present in cocoa) are antioxidant plant metabolites that belong to the family of flavonoids. In experimental studies involving breast cancer cell lines, epigallocatechin gallate (EGCG), the major catechin in green tea, has been shown to suppress cell viability, induce apoptosis,[36] and inhibit angiogenesis by reducing expression of vascular endothelial growth factor (VEGF).[37]

Green tea consumption appears to be especially valuable in decreasing the risk of prostate cancer.[38] Daily green tea intake specifically helps men with pre-cancerous prostate lesions reduce their risk of developing cancer by 90 percent.[39]

Caffeine in green tea may cause insomnia and aggravate inconti-
nence. Very high doses of caffeine can accelerate heart rate and raise
blood pressure. All caffeine-containing products can be habit-forming.
Caffeine easily crosses the placenta, so large amounts of green tea
should not be consumed by pregnant women. Caffeine also goes into
breast milk. There is a report of large amounts of green tea reducing
the blood-thinning effects of warfarin (Coumadin). This is because
green tea contains vitamin K.

VITAMIN C AND CANCER

Vitamin C (ascorbic acid) is an essential nutrient mostly recognized for
protecting the body from oxidative stress (harmful effects from highly
reactive free radicals) by its antioxidant action. However, there are other
very important functions of vitamin C, specially its role as a cofactor in
the formation of important body substances such as collagen. Vitamin
C accelerates reactions in biosynthetic pathways by activating enzymes
to which it donates electrons. The formation of collagen is dependent
on vitamin C because it helps put together several amino acids in its
structure. Collagen is the most abundant protein in mammals, making
up about 25 percent of the whole-body protein content. Collagen fibers
are a major body component that support most tissues and give cells
their structure. Strong collagen may help retard metastasis.

Ascorbic acid concentrates in white blood cells, which are in charge
of your immune defense against infections. Vitamin C also seems to
increase production of lymphocytes, the white cells important in anti-
body production and in coordinating cellular immune functions. Vitamin C may help you fight bacterial, viral, and fungal diseases. Taken in
higher dosages, ascorbic acid may actually increase interferon production and thus activate the immune response to viruses. Vitamin C also
participates in the formation of several neurotransmitters and hormones. The multiplicity of actions of vitamin C in the body might
explain the variety of effects that have been observed in some patients:
improved appetite and sleep, increased energy, less pain, and a feeling
of general well-being.

Vitamin C has been neglected as an ergogenic aid and in the treatment of many diseases (the common cold, cardiovascular disease, and cancer), mainly because of the lack of knowledge of ascorbate's biochemical and physiological functions when given in large doses. Ascorbic acid not only possesses antioxidant and pro-oxidant activities but also exhibits cytotoxic effects at higher concentrations.[40] Ascorbate in high doses inhibits mediators of inflammation (prostaglandins), which have been correlated with increased cell proliferation.[41] Also, a growth inhibitory effect has been produced by ascorbate or its derivatives in at least seven types of tumor cells.[42]

Vast literature exists on vitamin C and cancer. As early as 1949, ascorbate use was proposed for cancer therapy.[43] In 1952, it was proposed as a chemotherapeutic agent.[44] Hundreds of studies (in vitro, cell, animal, and human studies) have been published on this topic.[45] Long-term human studies have shown that vitamin C dietary supplements, when used in conjunction with other antioxidants, can reduce the risk of developing cancer.[46] Similar results were found for cancers of the prostate[47] and lung.[48]

Controversy over Vitamin C

The classical controversy on the role of vitamin C and cancer emerged in the late 1970s between the Linus Pauling Institute and the Mayo Clinic.[49] The Mayo Clinic studies did not replicate the Pauling Institute's positive results. The reality was that the studies were not done the same way: the Mayo Clinic studies only used one-time oral doses, while the Pauling Institute used multiple oral doses in addition to intravenous doses. We now know from the work of the National Institutes of Health (NIH) researchers in the 1990s that oral doses cannot reach the plasma vitamin C concentrations needed to achieve anti-cancer activity.

Another more recent controversy ensued with vitamin C and conventional cancer treatment. There has been a concern that vitamin C might reduce the effectiveness of chemotherapy and radiation by reducing the potency of the free radicals necessary for killing the cancer cells. This misconception was due in part to a study from Memorial Sloan-Kettering in 1999 in which they described how cancer cells acquire and concentrate vitamin C.[50] The researchers suggested that these intracellular concentrations of ascorbate may provide malignant cells with a "metabolic advantage." This published suggestion has been embraced by most medical practitioners without any questioning or further evaluation, although no data demonstrating this suggestion has been published. On the contrary, NIH studies and others have demonstrated that vitamin C, when used at high doses, is selectively toxic to cancer cells due to the generation of hydrogen peroxide, which will inhibit tumor growth.[51]

Pro-oxidant activity exhibited by vitamin C is probably the main mechanism by which it inhibits cancerous growth and metastasis. Its role as an energy intermediate is a possible secondary anti-cancer mechanism.[52] Physiologically, ascorbic acid provides electrons for enzymes and other electron acceptors. It is interesting that dead tissue has a full complement of electrons, while living tissue maintains a deficit of electrons. This shows how vitamin C is so necessary for life. Vitamin C assures a continuing electron exchange among body tissues, cell mitochondria, and molecules. All body functions are directly controlled and regulated by this physiological flow of electrons. This flow of electricity through the body also establishes and maintains the subtle, and still poorly understood, magnetic fields in the body that appear to be involved in maintaining the healthy state. A greater amount of vitamin C in the body enhances the flow of electricity, optimizing the ability of the cells to maintain aerobic energy production and metabolic intermediaries that facilitates cell communication. Disease exists when this flow is impaired, and death occurs when this flow stops. In support of this theory, it has been documented that osteoblast cells treated with ascorbic acid had a fourfold increase in respiration and a threefold increase in ATP production, which provided energy for cell differentiation.[53] Ascorbate in high concentrations may provide the high-energy electrons necessary for aerobic metabolism, a redox activity which may be important not only in mitochondria energy production but in the regulation of cell growth as well.[54]

Since the 1970s, in 280 peer-reviewed studies, including 50 human studies involving 8,521 patients (5,081 of whom were given nutrients), results have consistently shown that non-prescription antioxidants and other nutrients do not interfere with therapeutic modalities for cancer.

In fact, they enhance the effectiveness of these therapies, decrease their side effects, and protect normal tissues. In 15 human studies, 3,738 patients who took non-prescription antioxidants and other nutrients actually had increased survival.[55] None of the trials gave evidence of significant decreases in efficacy from antioxidant supplementation during chemotherapy.

Vitamin C Dosing

Studies have demonstrated that 60 mg of vitamin C a day can prevent scurvy. Obviously, this is not the optimal physiological dose. High blood vitamin C levels are associated with a low risk for cardiovascular disease and for certain types of cancer and other diseases. For such preventive function, it appears that a dose of at least 500 mg per day is adequate. However, when dealing with an existing cancer, we are not interested in reducing risk but in creating an environment to strengthen the body while inhibiting tumor cell growth. Any trauma or disease is a stress that will increase vitamin C requirements; the physical and emotional stress of cancer is no exception. So, how much do we need to help the body deal with these stressors in addition to fighting the disease? If we look into the animal kingdom, we will find a hint to answer that question.

Almost all mammals are able to synthesize vitamin C in their livers in a considerable amount and they can increase its production when there is a higher demand. Irwin Stone, Ph.D., (1907–1984) was one of the earliest scientists to realize vitamin C's potential. He postulated that primates lost the ability to synthesize vitamin C around 25 million years ago. If we use other species as a guide to calculate the amount of vitamin C that an average human should produce, adjusted to an equivalent body weight for humans under normal circumstances, it should be an average of 5,400 mg. Even though some may require more vitamin C to achieve maximum benefit, a practical dosing recommendation that is well tolerated by most people ranges between 3,000–5,000 mg per day.

The concentrations of vitamin C toxic to cancer cells can be achieved clinically by intravenous administration. Studies done with cell cultures suggest that in order to kill tumor cells, plasma concentrations should be around 400 mg/dL, which would require dozens of grams adminis-tered intravenously. While these doses are usually well tolerated, there are nutrients such as lipoic acid that when used simultaneously with vitamin C can maintain its killing effect at lower concentrations. If your health-care provider needs information about the application of high-dose intravenous vitamin C, please refer to the following publication: Riordan, H.D., R.B. Hunninghake, N.H. Riordan, et al. "Intravenous Ascorbic Acid: Protocol for Its Application and Use." *P R Health Sci J* 22:2 (2003): 225–232.

Safety/Toxicity of Vitamin C

Vitamin C is remarkably safe. When used in very large oral doses, it may cause gastrointestinal (GI) distress (gas, heartburn, nausea, or diar-rhea). Interestingly enough, it has been reported that patients with viral illnesses tend to increase their bowel tolerance to vitamin C. For peo-ple who are susceptible to GI distress, there are a variety of dosage forms that are gentle on the stomach, such as vitamin C with chelated minerals, buffered, and a liposomal preparation.

A genetic condition that results in inadequate levels of the enzyme glucose-6-phosphate dehydrogenase (G6PD) can cause sufferers to develop anemia after ingesting specific oxidizing substances, such as very large dosages of vitamin C. So, a laboratory test for G6PD defi-ciency is a must for patients interested in intravenous vitamin C.

Finally, a word on kidney stones and vitamin C. There is no evidence that vitamin C causes kidney stones, and therefore restriction of high-er doses of vitamin C for this reason is unwarranted. In a study of 45,251 men, doses of vitamin C above 1.5 grams actually reduced the risk of kidney stones.[56] Another large-scale, prospective study followed 85,557 women for 14 years and found no evidence that vitamin C caus-es kidney stones.[57] There was no difference in the occurrence of stones between people taking less than 250 mg per day and those taking 1.5 grams or more. Moreover, vitamin C may reduce the pH of the urine, making it less likely to produce renal calculi. Nevertheless, good hydra-tion is always recommended.

CHAPTER 5

Energy for
Cancer Patients

"If you do what you've always done,
you'll get what you've always gotten."
—ANONYMOUS

All physiological and chemical processes in the body need energy. Each cell produces adenosine triphosphate (ATP), a form of short-term stored energy made from carbohydrates, in the mitochondria. The initial step in the process of producing energy from sugar is called glycolysis. Glycolysis does not require oxygen (anaerobic) and produces a small amount of energy. This is the most simple way of producing cellular energy. Rapidly growing malignant cells typically have glycolytic rates up to 200 times higher than normal tissues. This phenomenon was described in 1930 by Otto Warburg, who claimed that cancer was primarily caused by a dysfunction in mitochondrial metabolism, which disrupts normal gene expression leading to uncontrolled growth.[1]

The Krebs cycle (or citric acid cycle) is a series of enzymatic reactions that use oxygen for cellular respiration. It produces more energy per glucose molecule and occurs within the mitochondria (the "battery" of the cell). The Krebs cycle creates energy that is transferable to all systems in the body, but it is limited by the quantity of minerals, enzymes, and other reactants. The same is true for the third energy-producing process called oxidative phosphorylation, which releases energy by moving electrons from donors to acceptors, such as oxygen, in so-called reduction/oxidation (redox) reactions.

TAMING CANCER CELLS

The altered energy metabolism of tumor cells can provide a target for a nontoxic chemotherapy approach. An increased glucose consumption rate has been observed in malignant cells. The transformation of normal cells to malignant may be due to defects in the aerobic respiratory pathways. Oxygen by itself has an inhibitory action on malignant cell proliferation by interfering with anaerobic respiration (fermentation and lactic acid production). During cell differentiation (where cell energy level is high), there is increased cellular production of oxidants, which appear to stimulate changes in gene expression that may lead to a terminal differentiated state. This overcomes malignancy.

The failure to maintain high ATP production may be a consequence of oxidative inactivation of key enzymes, especially those related to the Krebs cycle and the electron transport system. A distorted mitochondrial function (transmembrane potential) may result. This aspect is suggestive of an important mitochondrial involvement in the carcinogenic process. In this respect, ascorbate (vitamin C) may serve a physiological function by providing reductive energy—the electrons necessary to direct energy pathways in the mitochondria. Interestingly, ascorbate has been detected in the mitochondria and also found to be regenerated internally there.[2]

Oxygen, the final electron acceptor, is of great importance to the ascorbate-induced cytotoxic action on cancer cell proliferation by interfering with anaerobic respiration (fermentation), a commonly used energy mechanism of malignant cells. It would be worth investigating the status of the mitochondria of malignant cells since this may be relevant to the origin of malignancy. A problem in electron transfer activity might well be coupled to defective mitochondria and vitamin C may help correct this problem.

Evidence continues to accumulate to support that energy intermediates produce benefit against cancer either by interacting directly with ascorbate (in redox reactions) or by improving aerobic metabolism in the mitochondria. Let's now expand on the evidence of some of these nutrients and cancer, particularly lipoic acid, coenzyme Q_{10}, and carnitine.

LIPOIC ACID

Lipoic acid (alpha-lipoic acid) is a sulfur-containing fatty acid antioxidant with metal-chelating and anti-glycation capabilities. *Chelate* means "to grab," and subsequently remove a toxic metal, such as mercury, from the body. *Anti-glycation* means preventing sugar molecules from binding with protein or fat molecules, as may occur with aging. Lipoic acid is active in both fat and water phases, unlike most antioxidants. This gives lipoic acid an unusually broad spectrum of antioxidant action. Lipoic acid is useful for recycling, and therefore extending, the functions of vitamins C and E, glutathione, and coenzyme Q_{10}.

The body routinely converts some alpha-lipoic acid to dihydrolipoic acid, an even more effective antioxidant against dangerous free radicals consisting of both oxygen and nitrogen, which play a role in many conditions.[3] Over the past decade, studies on lipoic acid have proliferated and there is increasing understanding to support the use of lipoic acid as a therapeutic agent for the prevention and treatment of various conditions, such as diabetes, atherosclerosis, ischemic injury, neuronal degeneration, radiation injury, and heavy metal poisoning.[4]

The claims of an anticarcinogenic effect for alpha-lipoic acid are threefold:

- Its capacity to scavenge free radicals, including the hydroxyl radical

- Its capacity to regenerate vitamin C

- Its cofactor function in aerobic ATP generation

The hydroxyl radical is involved in all stages of the cancer process (from stage I to metastasis) and lipoic acid may be of benefit no matter the stage. Lipoic acid down-regulates genes that cause cancer without leading to toxicity. In one study, laboratory-induced cancer cells absorbed lipoic acid to saturation and this increased the lifespan of rats by 25 percent.[5]

A study provided evidence that lipoic acid induces multiple cell-cycle checkpoint arrest in cancer cells. In other words, a cancer cell's "quality control" mechanism is sabotaged. This can mean that when a cancer cell tries to reproduce, it kills itself trying. Lipoic acid's ability to encourage apoptosis (programmed cell death) in cancer cells supports

its potential as a chemopreventive agent.[6] Alpha-lipoic acid was prefer-
entially toxic to leukemia cell lines, credited in part to the antioxidant's
ability to induce apoptosis. Lipoic acid also activated the enzyme caspase, which kills leukemia cells.[7] Other researchers showed that lipoic
acid acted as a potentiator, amplifying the anti-leukemic effects of vitamin D. It is speculated that lipoic acid delivers much of its advantage
by inhibiting the appearance of damaging cytokines, signaling proteins
that may be overactivated in some cancers.[8] Finding that lipoic acid can
differentiate between normal and leukemic cells creates the possibility
of new treatment strategies to slow or overcome the disease.[9]

Studies on cancer cell models suggest that the tumor-suppressive
effect of lipoic acid is related to programmed cell death.[10] It seems that
the induction of apoptosis is selectively exerted in cancer and transformed cell lines while being less active toward normal non-transformed cells.[11] This selectivity of alpha-lipoic acid for transformed cells
supports its potential use in the treatment of neoplastic disorders.[12]

Our findings indicate a novel pro-oxidant role of lipoic acid in inducing apoptosis through its regulation by the protein family Bcl-2, which
may be exploited for the treatment of cancer. In human leukemic T
cells, lipoic acid also potentiated Fas-mediated apoptosis through redox
regulation without affecting normal cells from healthy humans.[13]

Lipoic acid recycles vitamin C and it also improves mitochondrial
function. A study reported that when lipoic acid is used simultaneously with vitamin C, the concentration of vitamin C required to kill 50
percent of tumor cells decreased by over 80 percent (from 700 mg/dL
to 120 mg/dL).[14] The researchers concluded that it would be feasible
to obtain this concentration by intravenous infusion and urged further
work to investigate the use of a combination of vitamin C and lipoic
acid as an anti-cancer agent. Another study demonstrated that lipoic
acid can effectively induce apoptosis in human colon cancer cells by a
pro-oxidant mechanism that is initiated by an increased uptake of oxygen radicals into mitochondria.[15]

Reduction of Chemotherapy Toxicity

Questions continually arise about using antioxidants, such as lipoic acid, with chemotherapy. Animal studies have found that alpha-lipoic acid decreased side effects associated with chemotherapy without decreasing the effectiveness of the drugs.[16] Another study combined use of alpha-lipoic acid and doxorubicin and this resulted in marginally increased survival of mice with leukemia.[17] In spite of this, coupling antioxidants with orthodox cancer therapy remains a complex issue that must take into consideration the type of malignancy and the drugs used.

Lipoic acid may protect from hearing loss and deafness produced by cisplatin. It is thought that free radicals produced by cisplatin attack the inner ear, while lipoic acid works by boosting levels of the antioxidant glutathione.[18] Lipoic acid effectively prevented a decrease in renal antioxidant defense system and prevented it in conjunction with cisplatin therapy.[19] Studies have also demonstrated that lipoic acid is beneficial in reducing side effects (specifically, cardiac toxicity) of cancer chemotherapy.[20]

Treatment with lipoic acid one day prior to Adriamycin administration maintained near normal enzyme activity and significantly reduced lipid peroxidation, proving it to be an effective cytoprotectant.[21] A small study found that alpha-lipoic acid given intravenously once a week for 3–5 weeks followed by oral doses three times a day was able to counteract cumulative oxaliplatin-related neuropathy.[22]

Safety/Toxicity and Dosing

Lipoic acid appears to have no significant side effects at dosages up to 1,800 mg daily.[23] Even intravenous administration has been documented to be safe in a trial involving twenty patients with type 2 diabetes, who received intravenous injections of 500 mg per day for ten days.[24] Animal studies have documented a high safety limit for lipoic acid; doses up to 60 mg per kilogram of body weight did not show any adverse event in studies that lasted two years.[25]

The dose for lipoic acid supplementation will depend on the type of lipoic acid and its intended use. The doses of oral lipoic acid used in several studies for treating complications of diabetes are between 300 and 600 mg daily.[26] Based on the study that documented the synergy between vitamin C and lipoic acid to increase malignant cell cytotoxicity, the dose of lipoic acid should typically be between 300 and 900 mg per day, divided in two or three doses.[27]

COENZYME Q_{10}

A coenzyme is a vitamin-like substance needed for the proper functioning of an enzyme. Coenzyme Q_{10} (coQ_{10} or ubiquinone) is the coenzyme for at least three mitochondrial enzymes responsible for accepting electrons in the aerobic energy production in the cell. CoQ_{10} is found in small amounts in a wide variety of foods (organ meats, natural vegetable oils, fish, nuts, spinach, broccoli, eggs, butter, wheat germ, and garlic) and is also synthesized in all tissues. It is present in most human cells, except in those with no mitochondria, such as the red blood cells and eye lens cells. The manufacture of coQ_{10} in the body requires eight vitamins and other trace elements (including vitamins B_6, C, B_2, and B_{12}, as well as folic acid, niacin, and pantothenic acid). Since coQ_{10} is necessary for cell respiration, a deficiency could disrupt normal cellular functions.

Blood coenzyme Q_{10} concentrations are not routinely monitored, but its decrease is associated with a variety of problems that deal ultimately with cell energy. Research has demonstrated that coQ_{10}'s antioxidant properties and its role in mitochondrial energy production makes it useful as an adjunct therapy for cardiovascular diseases (congestive heart failure, hypertension, stable angina, drug-induced cardiotoxicity, ventricular arrhythmia) and non-cardiac conditions (cancer, periodontal disease, compromised immune system, obstructive lung disease, muscular dystrophy).[28] In addition it can also be used effectively to prevent or treat adverse effects from the cholesterol-lowering agents known as statins.[29]

CoQ_{10} is necessary for DNA to replicate, and deficiencies could produce abnormalities affecting the genes controlling differentiation.[30] Researchers have found lower levels of coenzyme Q_{10} in the blood of patients with cancers of the breast, lung, and pancreas.[31] The mean plasma levels of coQ_{10}, along with alpha-tocopherol and gamma-tocopherol (forms of vitamin E), were significantly lower in patients with cervical neoplasia and cancer compared with controls.[32] One U.S. study compared twenty-seven women with normal Pap smears to seventy-five women with cervical cancer and cervical intraepithelial neoplasia. Women with cervical cancer and neoplasia had lower concentrations of cervical/vaginal cell coQ_{10} and vitamin E compared to women with normal Pap smears.[33] An observational study found that individuals with lung, pancreas, and especially breast cancer were more likely to have low plasma coenzyme Q_{10} levels than healthy controls.[34]

Twenty-one breast cancer patients underwent radical mastectomy for breast cancer. Coenzyme Q_{10} concentrations and antioxidant enzyme activities were measured in tumor and surrounding tumor-free tissues. Reactive oxygen species (free radicals) were increased in malignant cells, and it was postulated that this may cause overexpression of antioxidant enzymes and the consumption of coQ_{10}. Increased antioxidant enzyme activities may be related to decreased susceptibility of cells to carcinogenic agents and the response of tumor cells to the chemotherapeutic agents. Therefore, administration of coenzyme Q_{10} may induce a protective effect on breast tissue.[35]

In a study of thirty-two breast cancer patients with metastases to axillary lymph nodes, coenzyme Q_{10} plus high-dose antioxidant therapy (vitamins C and E, beta-carotene, selenium, and omega-3 and omega-6 fatty acids) were given in addition to conventional surgery and chemotherapy. During the eighteen-month study period, none of the patients showed signs of further metastases and six patients had partial tumor regression.[36] Continued follow-up on three of these six patients, with increased doses of coQ_{10}, documented remission throughout the 3–5 years of the study.[37]

Our findings suggest that baseline plasma coenzyme Q_{10} levels are a powerful and independent prognostic factor that can be used to estimate the risk for melanoma progression.[38] In addition to its anti-cancer effects, coQ_{10} has been found to have immune system–enhancing properties. Studies demonstrate recovery of human lymphocytes from oxidative DNA damage.[39] This can certainly help cancer patients have better resistance to viral infections.

Reduction of Chemotherapy Toxicity

Replacing enzymatic cofactors, such as coenzyme Q_{10}, can help alleviate the side effects of chemotherapy. Free radical damage can be reversed and mitochondrial functions preserved. Antioxidants can mitigate damage to normal tissues and reduce adverse effects without reducing the efficacy of chemotherapy.[40] CoQ_{10} may help reduce the toxic effects on the heart caused by daunorubicin and doxorubicin, two chemotherapy medications that are commonly used to treat a variety of cancers.[41]

Eighty-four breast cancer patients received a daily supplement of coenzyme Q_{10}, riboflavin, and niacin, along with tamoxifen twice a day. Breast cancer patients who took the supplement showed a significant reduction in cytokine levels, which may suggest a good prognosis and efficacy of treatment, and might even offer protection from metastases and recurrence of cancer.[42]

Studies in cells and animals, a few case reports, and an uncontrolled trial suggest that coQ_{10} supplementation may be beneficial as an adjunct to conventional therapy for breast cancer.[43] There is a need for controlled clinical trials to determine the effects of coenzyme Q_{10} supplementation in cancer patients.

Safety/Toxicity and Dosing

In one study, coenzyme Q_{10} was safe and well tolerated in thirty-one subjects treated with doses as high as 3,000 mg per day for eight months.[44] Oral administration of coQ_{10} improved subjective fatigue sensation and physical performance in healthy volunteers at doses of 300 mg.[45] In another study, coQ_{10} at doses of up to 900 mg did not cause any significant changes in symptoms or laboratory results as assessed by physical, hematological, blood biochemical, or urinalysis tests. Physician examinations also did not reveal any abnormalities.[46] Blood concentration of coQ_{10} decreases in patients receiving drug therapy with statin drugs, gemfibrozil, Adriamycin, and certain beta blockers. It seems logical to replace coQ_{10} in patients receiving these medications, given its safety and potential benefits.[47]

Coenzyme Q_{10} may decrease the effectiveness of blood-thinning medications such as warfarin, so coQ_{10} and blood-thinners should only be used together under careful medical supervision. In a study of individuals taking blood pressure medications (including diltiazem, metoprolol, enalapril, and nitrate), coQ_{10} supplementation allowed the individuals to take lower dosages.[48] This suggests that coQ_{10} may enhance the effectiveness of certain blood pressure medications or may have a hypotensive action, but more research is needed to verify these results.

The optimal dose of coenzyme Q_{10} will depend on individual needs. However, based on studies that used coQ_{10} successfully in cancer patients, typical doses between 100 and 400 mg should be adequate.[49] Following oral supplementation with the standard form of coQ_{10}, ubiquinone, most of it is reduced in the body to the usable form, ubiquinol. The ubiquinol form may be absorbed more efficiently than ubiquinone, increasing and maintaining higher blood levels.

CARNITINE

Carnitine is a derivative of the amino acids lysine and methionine. Its name is derived from the Latin word *carnus*, meaning "meat," from which it was first isolated. L-Carnitine is used in cells for the transport of fats from the cell fluid into the mitochondria for metabolic energy production, converting fatty acids into energy. Acetyl-L-carnitine is an acetylated form of L-carnitine—adding acetyl groups to molecules improves absorption—which can help repair the mitochondria, boost levels of important antioxidants such as glutathione and coenzyme Q_{10}, and work synergistically with lipoic acid.[50]

This compound is synthesized in the liver and kidneys and stored in the skeletal muscles, heart, brain, and sperm. Under certain conditions, the demand for this nutrient exceeds its production, making it a conditionally essential nutrient. Some people can have dietary deficiencies of carnitine or malabsorption of this nutrient. Genetic disorders as well as liver or kidney problems, high-fat diets, certain medications, and low dietary levels of the amino acids lysine and methionine can also lead to this problem.

Carnitine deficiencies may cause fatigue, chest pain, muscle pain, weakness, low blood pressure, and confusion. L-Carnitine has been used as a supplement in patients who have high cholesterol levels, and research has also indicated its use in cardiovascular disease, infertility, enhancement of athletic performance, and weight loss. Carnitine has shown value in the management of myocardial infarction, congestive heart failure, angina, and diabetes.[51]

Its role in cancer is currently being investigated and some of the benefits so far are related to improved quality of life and better tolerance of chemotherapy. It is postulated that when used along other mitochondrial-enhancing nutrients, it may help to revert the cancer process by facilitating energy production. Carnitine exerts a substantial antioxidant action, thereby providing a protective effect against oxidative stress induced at the cellular level. By facilitating aerobic respiration, carnitine could be important in transforming cell signaling toward a state of differentiation or apoptosis (programmed cell death).

In one cell culture study, L-carnitine was reported to have a different effect in normal and cancer cells. There were an increased number of dead liver cancer cells, while there was no difference in the number of normal cells. Messenger RNA and levels of TNF-alpha, Fas, and caspase-8, protein signals that are closely related to cell apoptosis, were increased by L-carnitine treatment. In addition, L-carnitine treatment regulated mitochondria-dependent apoptosis pathways.[52]

Reduction of Chemotherapy Toxicity

Fatigue is the most commonly reported symptom in patients with cancer, with a prevalence of over 60 percent reported in the majority of studies. Carnitine deficiency is a common and correctable cause of fatigue in cancer patients. L-Carnitine supplementation in patients with cancer, fatigue, and carnitine deficiency may be safely administered at doses up to 3,000 mg per day; positive effects may be more likely at relatively higher doses.

Another complication of chemotherapy is peripheral neurotoxicity, especially with agents such as platinum compounds, taxanes, and vinca alkaloids. Acetyl-L-carnitine is useful in the treatment of neuropathies.[53]

Safety/Toxicity and Dosing

At doses of approximately 3,000 mg per day, carnitine supplements may cause nausea, vomiting, abdominal cramps, diarrhea, and a "fishy" body odor. More rare side effects include muscle weakness in uremic patients and seizures in those with pre-existing seizure disorders. The evidence of safety is strong at doses up to 2,000 mg per day. Although much higher levels have been tested without adverse effects and may be safe, the data for intakes above 2,000 mg per day are not sufficient for a confident conclusion of long-term safety.[54]

Dietary supplementation with acetyl-L-carnitine is preferred because it is thought to be more bioavailable and biologically active. The typical dosing recommendation ranges from 500 to 1,000 mg daily. However, doses of up 1,000 mg three times a day may be needed for those with chemotherapy-induced neurotoxicity.

CHAPTER 6

Rejuvenation for Cancer Patients

"Progress is impossible without change, and those who cannot change their mind cannot change anything."
—GEORGE BERNARD SHAW (1856–1950)

In your one human lifetime, your eyes will blink 450 million times, you will breathe 650 million times, you will grow 1,000 layers of skin, your nails will grow 7 feet, you will lose 70 miles of hair from your head, and your heart will beat 2.5 billion times! If you rub your forearm briskly just for a few seconds, 300,000 skin cells will come off of it. By age seventy, you will shed 105 pounds of skin. If the total internal surface area of your stomach and intestinal tract were flattened out, it would be half the size of a regulation basketball court. There are seventy-two feet of nerves and nine feet of blood vessels for *every square inch* of your skin.

There are tens of trillions of cells in your body. *Every single one of them* is made from the nutrients you eat and drink. Not one cell in your body is made from a drug. If there were ever an argument for using abundant nutrients to rejuvenate an ailing body, this may be it.

IODINE

Iodine is the least reactive member of the family of elements called halogens. The term *halogen* means "salt former" and refers to a family that would like to pick up an electron, which makes them extremely active chemically. Iodinated compounds are essential for the normal growth and development of vertebrates. Iodide (a reduced form of iodine) functions as an antioxidant that can detoxify reactive oxygen species such as hydrogen peroxide. The thyroid gland actively accumulates iodide from the blood and incorporates it into thyroid hormones, which control the metabolic rates of many cells. Iodine is also found in breast tissue, adrenal glands, thymus, prostate, kidneys, liver, and intestines, among other organs.

Iodine is very important during gestation for both mother and child. Inadequate iodine intake during gestation results in irreversible damage to the fetal brain and the associated abnormally low thyroid hormone level in the mother. Iodine deficiency during pregnancy can produce neurological damage in the developing fetus.[1] The birth of many children with learning disabilities may be prevented by the use of iodine supplements, especially as part of the early prenatal care.

However, the role of iodine in the body goes far beyond its function in neurological development and thyroid hormone production. Other functions include helping to regulate moods, preventing cancer (especially in breasts, ovaries, uterus, prostate, and thyroid gland), preventing and treating fibrocystic breast disease in women, helping to regulate blood pressure and blood sugar (useful for preventing and treating diabetes), and preventing abnormal cardiac rhythms. Iodine functions as an antibacterial, antiviral, antiparasitic, and antifungal, and it also enhances immune function.[2]

Role in Cancer Therapy

Human breast tissue has an affinity for iodine. A deficiency of iodine has been linked with the development of fibrocystic breast disease (FBD or benign breast disease). Symptoms of FBD may include non-cancerous but painful lumps, enlarging cysts, breast nodules, and scar tissue. Generally, FBD happens in the premenstrual phase of a woman's cycle but it may involve the whole cycle. Menopausal women on estrogen therapy may also experience similar symptoms. More than 50 percent of women of reproductive age may have FBD, and many more women of all ages have been found to have fibrocystic disease–like changes at autopsy.[3] FBD has been identified as a risk factor for breast cancer.[4]

Diet has an important impact on breast health: vegetable fat, vitamin E, and fiber intakes during adolescence were inversely associated with risk of proliferative FBD. This may suggest a means for preventing breast cancer.[5] Sustained iodine depletion in animal studies not only produced benign changes but also produced breast cancer.[6] Iodine works by effectively reducing FBD,[7] with an important role in maintaining normal breast tissue architecture and function. Iodine may also have important antioxidant functions in breast tissue.[8]

Iodine may have a protective effect on breast cancer, although the exact mechanisms for this effect are still unknown. Evidence from clinical studies suggests that iodine may modulate the estrogen pathway. Researchers have identified genetic alterations (twenty-nine genes that were up-regulated, fourteen genes that were down-regulated) from iodine or iodide treatment, included genes involved in hormone metabolism, the cell cycle, growth, and differentiation. Thus, iodine/iodide may be useful as an adjuvant therapy for influencing the estrogen pathway in breast cancer.[9]

Iodine uptake into the cells occurs through a glycoprotein in the cell membrane called sodium-iodine symporter (NIS). Basal NIS genes are detected in about 80 percent of breast cancer specimens, but the number with functional iodide transport is low.[10] Higher levels of molecular iodine reduce the symptoms of mammary fibrosis, decrease mammary cancer induced chemically in rats, and have antiproliferative and apoptotic effects.[11] Animals receiving molecular iodine showed a reduction in mammary cancer. Iodine's proposed mechanism of action is reducing fat peroxidation in mammary glands, which is involved in carcinogenesis.[12]

The importance of these effects has been underestimated, in fear that high iodine doses could pose a risk to thyroid physiology. Besides the extensive experience of practitioners with the use of iodide, a recent study demonstrated that chronic iodine supplementation is not accompanied by any harmful secondary effects on the thyroid or on general health.[13] Therefore, iodine levels should be evaluated in cancer patients and its replacement should be considered. Considering its safety and potential benefits, we urge clinical trials to define the role of iodine in cancer.

Safety/Toxicity and Dosing

Selenium is required for the production of enzymes that regulate thyroid hormone availability and action. Clinical investigations have demonstrated that coexisting deficiencies (selenium and iodine) cause increased thyroid-stimulating hormone (TSH) levels and contribute to goiter development.[14] It is important to consider selenium supplementation to prevent potential thyroid damage from iodide supplementation in selenium-deficient individuals.[15]

The Recommended Dietary Allowance (RDA) for non-pregnant adults is 150 micrograms (mcg). Most unsupplemented diets contain less. However, Japanese women, who have one of the lowest breast cancer rates in the world, may ingest iodide amounts of over 13 mg (13,000 micrograms) of iodine daily from seaweed, without suffering any adverse effects. Doses of 3–6 mg (3,000–6,000 mcg) of molecular iodine taken for up to five years have been tested for treatment of breast pain and fibrosis in patients without pre-existing autoimmune thyroid pathologies. Therapeutic success was achieved in over 70 percent of the cases without manifestations of thyroid abnormalities.[16]

For cancer patients, the typical recommended dose is up to 25 mg (25,000 mcg) per day.

ENZYMES

Enzymes are proteins found in every cell of plants and animals. They are the catalysts of biochemical reactions—they accelerate reaction rates in living systems. There are over 3,000 different enzymes in the body, each of them performing a specific task and each working under unique conditions, such as a specific range of pH (acid/alkaline balance). Proteolytic enzymes digest only proteins, whereas the various pancreatic enzymes digest fats and starches. Enzymes stimulate chemical reactions in association with coenzymes or cofactors. Cofactors are substances that must be present for an enzyme to work efficiently (such as zinc, magnesium, or copper), while coenzymes are organic substances that combine with an inactive enzyme to form an active one.

Certain inhibitors in the body block the activity of enzymes and the production of enzymes can be decreased by disease, injury, stress, aging, and poor nutrition. If enzymes are decreased in the body, in order to function properly they must be acquired from an outside source.

Digestive enzymes (hydrolases) break down foods into smaller molecules making them easier to digest. Proteases are enzymes that break down proteins, amylases work on carbohydrates, and lipases lyse (break up) fats. The salivary glands, stomach walls, pancreas, liver, and intestines produce and dispense enzymes for digestion. Enzymes are also found in meats, fresh fruits, and vegetables in the diet. Enzymes from animal sources include trypsin, chymotrypsin, pepsin, rennin, and pancreatin. Enzymes from plants utilized in dietary supplements include bromelain (from pineapple), papain (from papaya), and malt diastase. Pineapple, papaya, kiwi, and ginger root are known to have high protease content as well. Finally, microbial enzymes are those produced by either fungi or bacteria, mainly through fermentation.

Beside their functions in facilitating chemical reactions such as digestion, enzymes have been found to have various activities against cancer cells. Our choices on how to eat can have a big impact on the reserves of pancreatic enzymes. When you eat diets high in protein and refined foods (meat, sugar, and white flour products), you deplete your pancreatic enzymes. Without enough pancreatic enzymes available to dissolve the protein coat of cancer cells that may be present in the body, cancer cells start getting protection (coating) and food (sugar). The proteolytic enzymes used in cancer studies usually consist of a combination of papain, trypsin, and chymotrypsin. Clinical studies have demonstrated that they are valuable in the management of cancer by improving quality of life and prolonging survival.

Role in Cancer Therapy

Scottish embryologist John Beard (1857–1924) was one of the pioneers in suggesting enzymes for treating cancer in the early 1900s. Dr. Beard observed that cells in the placenta, growing in preparation for the fetus, resemble malignant or cancerous cells. But the placental tissue ceases growth once pancreatic enzyme production begins in the fetus. From this, Dr. Beard theorized that pancreatic enzymes could also be used to halt the growth of malignant tumors.[17] Dr. Beard's idea inspired others, leading to the publication of several case reports documenting tumor regression and remission in terminal cancer patients using proteolytic enzymes.[18] Dr. Beard published a monograph in 1911 explaining his therapy and the supporting evidence,[19] but his ideas did not gain enough interest from the scientific and medical community at the time.

Forty years later, William Donald Kelley (1925–2005), a Texas dentist, used Dr. Beard's ideas to cure his own case of advanced pancreatic cancer. He used a protocol based on nutrition along with high-dose pancreatic enzymes and other supplements. After this success, he treated thousands of other "terminal" cancer patients. Despite clinical documentation of extraordinary results, it did not raise much interest among the medical community. Scientific evaluation of this natural, nontoxic treatment against cancer finally occurred when Nicholas Gonzalez, M.D., studied the results from Kelley's patients. He published a paper that demonstrated that patients with advanced pancreatic cancer had longer survival times when they used Kelley's approach.[20]

It is not exactly clear how enzymes provide these benefits, but the molecular action of enzymes against cancer cells is currently being investigated. The anti-inflammatory effect of systemic enzyme therapy seems to be one of the most important mechanisms of action. Oral enzyme supplementation affects adhesion molecules and produces alterations of cytokine composition, both of which impact immune response.[21] It may help reduce swelling and inflammation and activate macrophages, natural killer (NK) cells, and immune complexes.[22] Other proposed anti-cancer mechanisms include down-regulation of the immunosuppressive cytokine TGF-beta,[23] direct inhibition of tumor cell growth, and effects on platelet aggregation and thrombosis.

Cancer cells are commonly covered by a resistant sugar/protein coating (mucoprotein), which hides them from immune cells and may also protect them partially from chemotherapy. If we can strip the cancer tissue of that protection, the immune system cells may identify and mount a proper response; other therapeutic strategies can be more effective as well. Pancreatic enzymes, especially trypsin and chymotrypsin, are useful in dissolving the protein coat of the cancer cell, making it vulnerable to the attack of white blood cells.

The accumulation of fibrin/fibrinogen and other coagulation factors in and around solid tumors is an important aspect of the metastatic ability of cancer cells. The function of proteolytic enzymes in cancer treatment is to remove these factors that can protect or stimulate metastasis. Metastases involve a cascade of pathophysiological processes and are responsible for more than 60 percent of cancer deaths worldwide.[24] This means that if we can stop a tumor from producing metastasis, many deaths can be prevented. Pancreatic enzymes seem to be a helpful tool to control or prevent metastasis. Fibrin/fibrinogen may be involved in tumor growth and metastasis by forming a frame to which tumor cells can attach and a shelter to protect tumor cells from attack by activated lymphocytes; it may also help in the formation of new blood vessels in tumor tissues.[25]

In general, the immune system does not normally react to its own cells. However, when a cell becomes malignant, antigens form on the surface of the transformed cell. The immune system may then identify these cells as foreign and destroy them. But this does not occur all the time. In many instances, the antigens on the surface of cancer cells are surrounded with fibrin and mucous substances that make it difficult for the immune system to reach them and identify them as foreign. In a study on liver cell proliferation, the enzyme papain stimulated DNA synthesis and mitosis. It also showed that the cell coat mucopolysaccharide disappears temporarily in papain-treated animals, which may help the immune system recognize the cancer cell.[26] Findings in inhibiting metastasis using enzyme therapy given rectally have also been documented.[27]

In 1999, Dr. Gonzalez conducted a two-year, unblinded pilot study with ten patients suffering from pancreatic cancer (stages II to IV of the disease). The patients were treated with large doses of orally ingested pancreatic enzymes, resulting in an 81 percent survival rate of one year, 45 percent survival rate of two years, and 37 percent survival rate of three years.[28] Pancreatic cancer is a lethal disease with a poor survival rate in comparison with other diseases.[29] A study in mice with pancreatic cancer treated with pancreatic enzyme extracts showed that they survived significantly longer in comparison with the control group.[30] These data suggest an increase in survival rate due to the consumption of oral enzymes.

Oral enzymes such as bromelain have also been proposed as additive agents for conventional cancer therapy.[31] A retrospective cohort study using oral enzymes as a complementary treatment after breast cancer surgery showed improvement in the quality of life, a reduction in side effects from conventional therapies, and a prolongation in survival.[32] A similar study was conducted in patients with colorectal cancer, also showing longer survival times.[33] More research and clinical studies need to be done in order to better understand the mechanism of action of enzymes in cancer and their possible use as a treatment.

Safety/Toxicity and Dosing

Before taking pancreatic enzymes, tell your doctor if you are allergic to them or to pork protein, or if you have any other allergies. The therapeutic value of an enzyme is directly dependent on its activity, which is indicated in various units; however, there are no specific methods of measuring proteolytic enzymes. Enzyme consumption does not appear to have any long-term side effects because they are eliminated after 24–48 hours. Short-term side effects could include changes in the stool, gastrointestinal disturbances, and minor allergic reaction, all of them disappearing when therapy is discontinued.

Diarrhea, constipation, abdominal pain/cramps, nausea, or vomiting may occur. If any of these effects persist or worsen, tell your doctor promptly. Remember that your doctor has prescribed this medication because he or she has judged that the benefit to you is greater than the risk of side effects. Many people using enzymes do not have any serious adverse effects. Tell your doctor immediately if any of these rare, but serious, side effects occur: severe constipation, severe stomach/abdominal discomfort, frequent/painful urination, or joint pain.

Some studies have shown an adverse effect with trypsin in the prognosis and metastasis of certain cancers. In 2003, researchers conducted a study of trypsin expression in colorectal cancer and found that patients with trypsin-positive carcinoma had shorter and disease-free survival periods. Trypsin activates matrilysin, which has a role in colon cancer progression.[34] Trypsin may also activate matrix metalloproteinases

(MMPs) and epidermal growth factor receptor (EGFR), thus promoting tumor metastasis.[35]

Clinical studies with good results have used formulations that contained trypsin (40 mg), chymotrypsin (40 mg), and papain (100 mg), usually 2 tablets, three times a day. However, commercial products can vary substantially. A general recommendation is 4 tablets of a combination enzyme supplement, four times a day, two hours before or after food intake. If you have digestive problems, you may add 2–4 tablets with a meal. Antacids may decrease the effectiveness of pancreatic enzymes.

OMEGA-3 FATTY ACIDS

Essential fatty acids (EFAs) cannot be manufactured by the body. And, as Yogi Berra would say, "You don't have them, so that's why you need them." Specifically, you need to eat them. Saturated fatty acids contain only single carbon-carbon bonds. "Saturated" means they are full to capacity with hydrogen molecules. These are generally animal fats, but palm and coconut oils are also saturated. Unsaturated fatty acids have one or more carbon double bonds. Each of these could be opened up to grab more hydrogen molecules, therefore they are considered "unsaturated." Most vegetable oils are unsaturated.

Monounsaturated oils (one carbon double bond) include oleic acid, found in olives, peanuts, almonds, and avocados. Polyunsaturated fatty acids (two or more carbon double bonds) are more typical in vegetable oils. Omega-3 and omega-6 fatty acids are the two primary types. Most vegetable oils that you eat are omega-6 fatty acids, such as linoleic acid. There are three major types of omega-3 oils: alpha-linolenic acid (ALA), eicosapentaenoic acid (EPA), and docosahexaenoic acid (DHA). The body converts ALA to EPA and DHA, which are more readily used by the body.

Because they are EFAs, omega-3 fatty acids must be obtained from food. Omega-3 fatty acids can be found in fish (such as salmon, tuna, and halibut), other marine life (algae and krill), green leafy plants (especially purslane), seeds, whole grains, beans, nuts, and nut oils. It is important to maintain an appropriate balance of omega-3s and omega-6s in the diet, as these two substances work together to promote health. Omega-3s help reduce inflammation, and most omega-6s tend to promote inflammation. An imbalance of these EFAs contributes to the development of disease, while a proper balance helps maintain and even improve health. The healthiest of diets would consist of roughly equal amounts of omega-6 and omega-3 fatty acids. The typical American diet is incredibly far from that ideal, tending to contain 20 or even 40 times more omega-6s than omega-3s. This imbalance is a significant factor in the rising rate of inflammatory disorders. A 2:1 or even a 5:1 ratio would be a big improvement.

Omega-3 fatty acids help ameliorate the risk factors of chronic heart disease, cancer, and arthritis. They are also highly concentrated in brain tissue and are important for memory and behavioral functions of the brain. Deficiency symptoms include fatigue, memory/concentration difficulties, dry skin, mood swings, and heart and circulation problems. The omega-3 fatty acids are capable of regulating metabolic functions, affect gene expression, and help to reduce inflammation by inhibiting eicosanoid pathways.[36] Omega-3s incorporate into the cell membrane, making it more flexible, durable, and efficient.

Role in Cancer Therapy

The consumption of omega-3 fatty acids inhibits a number of mechanisms related to promotion and progression of tumors.[37] It has been implicated in reducing the production of certain hormones, such as estrogen, which is known to be a risk factor in breast cancer.[38] Consumption of omega-3 fatty acids replaces arachidonic acid in inflammatory cells with eicosapentaenoic acid, and therefore has an anti-inflammatory effect.[39] Omega-3s improve survival of cancer patients by reducing inflammation, suppressing mitosis, restoring functional apoptotic pathways (programmed cell death) to help control cancer growth, inducing cell differentiation, suppressing angiogenesis (blood vessel formation related to tumors), and altering estrogen metabolism.[40]

In a prospective, randomized, double-blind clinical trial with forty-four patients who had a major abdominal cancer surgery, it was found that fish oil supplementation improved liver and pancreas function, contributing to the patients' recovery.[41] Studies of omega-3 fatty acids in patients with prostate cancer suggest that it decreases the growth of prostate cancer cells by altering hormone activity.[42] Studies suggest that omega-3s have anti-tumor effects during initiation and post-initiation stages of colorectal cancer.[43]

In breast cancer, it has been shown that omega-3s are able to modulate protein kinase-A and protein kinase-C (enzymes involved with the metabolism of proteins), which are overexpressed in terminal cancer patients; this is reported to arrest the development of breast cancer. The oxidation of long-chain polyunsaturated fatty acids present in fish oil, such as EPA and DHA, can produce an array of lipid oxidation products that may possess cytostatic (inhibiting cell growth and cell division) or cytolytic (cell destroying) capacity.[44] This may be the main mechanism in controlling cancer.

Safety/Toxicity and Dosing

Omega-3 fatty acids are considered safe by the U.S. Food and Drug Administration (FDA). However, fish oil supplements may cause gastrointestinal problems, including potentially severe diarrhea at high doses. Other side effects include burping, heartburn, bloating, and abdominal pain. Side effects can be reduced if the fish oil is taken with food and if people start with lower dosages and only gradually increase them. Fish liver oil contains the fat-soluble vitamins A and D, and therefore fish liver oil products (such as cod liver oil) may increase the risk of vitamin A or D toxicity.

Omega-3s can contribute to an increased risk of bleeding (nosebleeds and blood in the urine), although lower doses are generally regarded as safe. It is thought that fish oils may decrease platelet aggregation, thus prolonging bleeding time, and increase the breaking down of blood clots. Theoretically, omega-3 fatty acids could increase bleeding risk when taken with certain drugs, such as blood thinners and NSAIDs, or with herbs and supplements such as *Ginkgo biloba*, garlic, and vitamin E.

Clinical trials have reported small dose-responsive reductions in blood pressure with omega-3 fatty acids. DHA may have a larger effect on blood pressure than EPA. So, caution is advised for people who have low blood pressure or who are taking drugs for high blood pressure.

Pregnant women, nursing mothers, young children, and women who might become pregnant should not eat several types of fish, including swordfish, shark, and king mackerel, because of concerns over heavy metal contamination (such as mercury). These individuals should also limit consumption of other fish, including albacore tuna, salmon, and herring. Most safety concerns apply to eating fish but likely not to ingesting fish oil supplements.

There is no Recommended Dietary Allowance (RDA) for omega-3 fatty acids, but you should try to get at least 1 gram a day.

VITAMIN D

Vitamin D is fat-soluble and is naturally present in a few foods; it is also manufactured by the body when sunlight strikes the skin. Vitamin D must be converted to an active form in the body: first in the liver to 25-hydroxyvitamin D (calcidiol) and second in the kidney to 1,25-dihydroxyvitamin D (calcitriol). Vitamin D is essential for calcium absorption and for maintaining adequate calcium and phosphate concentrations for bone mineralization. Without sufficient levels of vitamin D in the body, bones may become brittle or misshapen. Vitamin D helps prevent rickets in children and, together with calcium, also helps protect older adults from osteoporosis. In regard to cancer, genes involved in cell proliferation, differentiation, and apoptosis are affected by vitamin D. It targets a variety of genes throughout the body and thus has many mechanisms of action. One meta-analysis of clinical trials found that taking cholecalciferol (vitamin D_3) significantly reduced mortality.[45] Deficiency has been implicated in many of the chronic diseases of civilization.

Role in Cancer Therapy

In a four-year, double-blind, randomized, placebo-controlled trial involving thousands of healthy postmenopausal women, it was found that improving calcium and vitamin D nutritional status through supplementation substantially reduced all-cancer risk in the women.[46] Calcium and vitamin D both appear to have antineoplastic effects in the large bowel. Although these nutrients are interrelated metabolically in bone and in the normal intestine, their potential interactions in large-bowel carcinogenesis are not well understood. Normal supplemental doses of vitamin D are associated with decreases in mortality rates from all causes, but the relationship among baseline vitamin D status, supplement dose, and mortality rates needs to be investigated.[47] Calcium supplementation and vitamin D status appear to act largely together, not separately, to reduce the risk of colorectal adenoma recurrence.[48] The evidence to date suggests that daily intake of 1,000–2,000 IU per day of vitamin D could reduce the incidence of colorectal cancer.[49]

Safety/Toxicity and Dosing

Vitamin D deficiency can be addressed by using sunlight (or artificial ultraviolet radiation) or vitamin D_3 supplementation. A typical dose for a healthy person is 2,000–7,000 IU of vitamin D per day. However, those with illnesses associated with vitamin D deficiency—cancer, heart disease, multiple sclerosis, diabetes, autism—should probably supplement at higher levels, supervised by a physician. Vitamin D supplement doses higher than government recommendations (200–600 IU) may lead to better health. However, the optimum serum concentrations of vitamin D have not been delineated. For bone health, increasing the recommended intake of vitamin D is critical. A daily intake of 1,000 IU of cholecalciferol is the minimal amount needed for optimum health; 1,500–2,000 IU might lead to greater improvement.[50]

A general therapeutic recommendation is 5,000 IU of vitamin D daily.

PROBIOTICS

Probiotics are "pro life" as opposed to antibiotics that are against it. Specifically, this is about "good" bacteria versus "bad" bacteria. Friendly bacteria are present in many foods, such as yogurt. *Lactobacillus* and *Bifidobacteria* strains are most frequently used as probiotic supplements to promote healthy function of the gastrointestinal tract. Many investigators have evaluated the therapeutic effects of probiotics against diseases such as cancer, infections, and gastrointestinal disorders. An increase in immune cell activity has been described, and another possible explanation for the health benefits of probiotics may be their effect on other bacteria in the intestine. Probiotics may suppress the growth of bacteria that convert pro-carcinogens into carcinogens, thereby reducing the amount of carcinogens in the intestine.[51]

Role in Cancer Therapy

Dysregulation of the microflora in the gut can lead to inflammatory disorders and eventually also to cancer.[52] Although a myriad of health-promoting effects have been attributed to probiotic bacteria, perhaps the most interesting and controversial is that of anti-cancer activity, the vast majority of studies in this area dealing with protective effects against colon cancer. *Lactobacillus acidophilus* may potentially prevent colon cancer development; further studies are warranted to determine the full potential of this probiotic.[53] Probiotic supplementation reduces the biological effects of aflatoxin (a poison from food contaminated with toxic fungi *Aspergillus flavus* and *A. parasiticus*) exposure and may thereby offer an effective dietary approach to decrease the risk of liver cancer.[54] *Lactobacillus* supplementation may reduce the frequency of severe diarrhea and abdominal discomfort related to chemotherapy.[55] There is no direct experimental evidence for cancer suppression in humans as a result of the consumption of probiotic cultures in fermented or unfermented foods, but there is a wealth of indirect evidence, based largely on laboratory studies.[56]

Safety/Toxicity and Dosing

There are no safety issues with probiotics. Some temporary bloating or gas may occur at the start of use. This resolves quickly as the probiotic's good bacteria displace the bad bacteria.

Recommended general dose of a probiotic is 2–4 billion live organisms at least once a day. That is usually just a matter of several capsules or tablets.

VITAMIN K

Vitamin K is necessary for normal clotting of blood in humans; specifically, it is required for the liver to make factors necessary for blood to properly clot (coagulate). Deficiency of vitamin K or disturbances of liver function (for example, severe liver failure) may lead to deficiencies of clotting factors and excess bleeding. Vitamin K_1 (phytonadione) is the natural form of vitamin K, which is found in plants (such as broccoli, kale, Swiss chard, alfalfa, and parsley) and provides the primary source of vitamin K to humans through the diet. Vitamin K_2 compounds (menaquinones) are made by bacteria in the human gut and provide a smaller amount of one's vitamin K requirement. Vitamin K_3, menadione, is a synthetic form, which your body can make into K_2. However, K_3 is not nearly as safe as the other forms.

While vitamin K deficiency is rare these days, it should be of concern because it can cause abnormalities in blood clotting and thus increased bleeding. Deficiency may be found in those with chronic malnutrition (including alcohol dependency) or people with conditions that limit dietary absorption (such as celiac disease, ulcerative colitis, or cystic fibrosis). Drugs such as antibiotics, salicylates, anti-seizure medications, and sulfa drugs may reduce vitamin K absorption.

Role in Cancer Therapy

In one study, vitamin K_3 diminished cell viability and arrested the cell cycle in the G_2/M phase in a dose-dependent manner. It significantly enhanced the cytotoxicity of etoposide, an anti-cancer agent, and reduced the cytotoxic activity of irinotecan, an S phase–dependent agent. These findings suggest that vitamin K_3 induces G_2/M arrest and is thus useful as an enhancer of G_2 phase–dependent drugs in liver cancer chemotherapy.[57] Administration of vitamin K_2 to mice inoculated with liver tumor cells reduced both tumor growth and body weight loss.[58] The results indicate that vitamins K_2 and K_3 may be useful agents for the treatment of patients with liver cancer.[59] Several studies have also shown a role for vitamin K in inducing apoptosis (programmed cell death) in cancer cells.[60]

Safety/Toxicity and Dosing

The blood-thinning drug warfarin inhibits vitamin K–dependent clotting factors. It is used for atrial fibrillation, artificial heart valves, and clotting disorders (hypercoagulability). Since vitamin K can decrease warfarin's blood-thinning effects, people on warfarin should avoid foods high in vitamin K as well as vitamin K supplements.

Recommended general dose is 45 mg of vitamin K_2 per day.

CHAPTER 7

Patient Success Stories

"The person who says it cannot be done
should not interrupt the one doing it."
—CHINESE PROVERB

Fresh out of college, I (Andrew) lived up in the hills of Vermont. My elderly friend Maurice, an octogenarian of French-Canadian extraction, and I were talking one day. I was twenty-something, with two toddlers. I said to him, very facetiously, "Maurice, I'm getting old." He thought about that for a spell, giving it far more consideration than it was worth. Presently the old gentleman answered, with a childish grin: "Keep right on!"

I took that to mean that if you keep right on getting older, you are still here. I mean, consider the alternative! Remember the teaching of one of history's great yogis (Yogi Berra): "It ain't over 'til it's over."

While there is life, there is much more than hope alone. Namely:

- A condition may be serious, and generally considered fatal by expert medical opinion; well, expert opinion has been wrong before this. Dewey did not defeat Truman.

- Health practitioners often hide from patients when they think nothing more can be done. Too bad, because many patients work harder when their back is against the wall. Harness that will to live and go for it. Death is to be denied, fought, and beaten for as long as possible. There is too much talk about "preparing for death," "putting affairs in order," and "accepting death as a fact of life." You can if you want, but I will never negotiate with death. Death is described as the "last enemy" in the Bible. We're all going to go, but we certainly don't have to go quietly. Life may be fatal to everyone, but it doesn't have to be today and it doesn't have to be you. Don't wait until you hear the rattle of death; duck and run for it now. Is this an attitude of "denying" death? Not really. When I was in Africa, we did not deny the existence of cobras or lions when we avoided them. Keep fighting, and don't worry about hurting death's feelings by doing it.

• Aggressive use of vitamins and radical diet revision most definitely have their place in the science of therapeutics. If you are really sick, and still haven't tried these, then you haven't lived yet. Know about nutrition and vitamin therapies and all possible options. Never say never, and do your homework. Were he a physician, Will Rogers might have said "All I know is what I read in the journals." Get your nose out of the *Journal of the American Medical Association* and read other journals, such as the *Journal of Orthomolecular Medicine*.

• If your doctor is "too busy" to seriously investigate alternatives, then find someone else. It only takes half a minute for a physician to provide a patient with an alternative medicine reading list and the suggestion, "Take vitamins, eat a plant-based diet, get and use a juicer, and load up on vitamin C." We insist that these are very potent and very low-risk additional measures. We do not trivialize medicine nor do we guarantee miracles when we urge full use of alternatives. Doctors and patients alike must do everything possible to get well. Every physician is duty bound to offer all options "for the good of the patient, to the best of my ability."

• All three of us have worked with the seriously ill and have come into intensive care units to find beds empty that yesterday contained a friend. Sometimes it was because he'd died during the night; sometimes it was because she went home well. No one knows how long they have to live, whether sick or not.

Should you be afraid that it might be too late for you, remember this: some 98 percent of the atoms in your body are replaced every year. Just think: very nearly all of you is brand new every twelve months. And every one of those atoms can only come from what you breathe, drink, and eat. Now there is one final reason to improve your diet and lifestyle. Here are some people who did:

LUNG CANCER

R.J., 55, is an Army veteran with a history of chronic smoking associated with chronic obstructive pulmonary disease (COPD). In 2002, he was evaluated for a lung mass with a positron emission tomography (PET) scan, and it suggested malignancy. At the same time, his younger sister, C.J., also a heavy smoker, was diagnosed with a similar lung malignancy. R.J. consulted us and decided to follow our experimental protocol (intravenous vitamin C, a vegetarian diet, and the regimen of supplements suggested in this book) in addition to conventional treatment, while C.J. decided to follow the conventional treatment alone. After following the RECNAC II protocol, his COPD improved to a point that he did not need medication and he could walk two miles without needing oxygen, a feat not possible for the previous three years! R.J. had a stable PET scan for nearly two years when he decided to have surgery. His sister was not so fortunate: C.J. died after six months of conventional therapy. R.J. retired and is doing well.

SKIN CANCER

H.E., 51, is a massage therapist who was diagnosed with squamous cell carcinoma of the face. Radiation therapy was recommended but she decided to undergo intravenous vitamin C therapy, beginning in March 2007. She receiving intravenous vitamin C once a week, used oral supplements in addition, and modified her diet to emphasize high-fiber, low-sugar, whole foods and eliminate junk food. H.E. was re-evaluated by her dermatologists in July and they stated that there was absolutely no sign of skin cancer and that she was looking better than before. She has completed six months of intravenous therapy and she is thrilled not only because her cancer has gone away, but because her skin complexion is great after the vitamin C treatment.

BREAST CANCER

In 2006, R.R., 47, was diagnosed with an invasive breast cancer, regionally advanced (two tumors, 3.5 and 2.7 cm) with lymph node involvement. Given the aggressiveness and advanced stage of her condition and the poor prognosis in standard protocols, her oncologist recommended that she enter an experimental protocol with ten other patients. Frightened by her diagnosis, she called us for advice and recommendations. We patiently explained our research and what we would do if we had cancer. We took great care, as always, to avoid robbing her of the precious gift of hope.

R.R. received our oral supplementation protocol before, during, and after an aggressive chemotherapy treatment that started in June 2006. The experimental chemotherapy was so intense that only two patients were able to tolerate it with good quality of life. These two patients were the only ones that followed the RECNAC II oral supplementation protocol. In October, she had breast surgery and reconstruction.

She had requested to the surgeon that a pathologist be present in the operating room to determine if breast removal was absolutely necessary. On the day of the surgery, she asked if the pathologist would be present and was reassured that he would. Unfortunately, no pathologist was present, and the surgeon removed the breast. Contrary to all expectations, there were no cancer cells found in the breast tissue removed. The surgeon was extremely surprised, because according to the cancer literature and his own experience, there is always residual cancer despite the most aggressive chemotherapy.

R.R. recovered from surgery quickly and returned to work in a few months. But the failure to respect her request of a pathologist, and deceiving her about it, took a heavy emotional toll. During the process of reconstruction, she suffered enormous emotional and physical pain, as well as complications that lasted over a year. Deep pain takes time and support to heal. Physically, she is doing great: all her tests are fine, she looks wonderful, and she is physically very active. This experience had a profound impact on R.R.: it gave her an opportunity to reevaluate not only her diet and supplementation but also other aspects of her life. She now has renewed inner strength and is in greater command of her life's journey.

L.W., 54, is a banker who was diagnosed with infiltrative carcinoma of the left breast in December 2007. Given the aggressiveness of the lesion, she was recommended to immediately start with chemotherapy. She had heard about RECNAC II, but at the time was unable to contact us. In January 2008, she received her first chemotherapy with Adriamycin and cyclophosphamide. She immediately experienced secondary effects such as hair loss, generalized weakness, change in coloration of skin, dizziness, and a marked decrease in blood count.

A week later, she started with RECNAC II protocol and saw an immediate improvement. Hair loss diminished immediately (she never lost her eyelashes or eyebrows), skin and nail color improved, she continued working regularly, there was no need for use of anti-emetics, and she discontinued the use of medication to increase blood count.

In April, after her third chemotherapy treatment, L.W. had a second magnetic resonance imaging (MRI) scan, which revealed a marked reduction in the size of the tumor, a situation that impressed her radiologist and oncologist. To date, she continues on the RECNAC II protocol and feels extremely well physically, emotionally, and spiritually. She has felt so well with the vitamin C protocol that she considers this should be administered to all cancer patients. She understands that to date there is no definitive cure for cancer, that there are many factors involved, and that you should treat them all—emotional, physical, and spiritual. She changed her lifestyle and is enjoying life to its maximum.

I.M., 55, is a physician who was diagnosed with invasive (stage III–IV) carcinoma of the left breast at age 49. Her prognosis was poor. She was immediately recommended routine chemotherapy, radiation therapy, a research protocol, and five years of Tamoxifen, an estrogen modifier. Her oncologist felt the case was too advanced and on each of her visits all he would do was scratch his head.

I.M. was a single parent with a ten-year-old son and an eighteen-year-old daughter who had just started college, so she knew she had to do whatever she could to survive. She immediately had a lumpectomy performed. Chemotherapy was delayed until she was accepted to participate in a research protocol, but she started with a round of Adriamycin with cyclophosphamide and then Taxotere, an anti-mitotic drug. She lost twenty pounds and was not looking or feeling good. I.M. was then scheduled to start on thirty-six sessions of radiation therapy.

In the meantime, she had been looking for alternative treatments and was informed of a protocol in Colombia that consisted of intravenous vitamin C and homeopathic medication. With her poor prognosis and her life at stake, I.M. decided to give it a try. She informed her oncologist that before starting radiation she wanted to travel to Colombia to seek an alternative treatment, and he told her that it was not a good decision. Despite this, she traveled to Colombia, stayed at a clinic for a couple of weeks, and received treatment. She then heard about physicians in Medellin, Colombia, who where performing energy medicine treatments with great results, so she decided to give that a try as well.

After completing these treatments, I.M. had an inner feeling that she was actually healed. She returned to Puerto Rico, spoke with the oncologists, and told them that she was not going to have any additional treatments. Disappointed and upset, they said she was putting her life at risk. I.M. continued seeking alternative treatments in Colombia, Mexico, and El Salvador, until she discovered that we were offering these protocols at the University of Puerto Rico. We started working with her.

I.M. has now entered her seventh year of remission, is cancer free, and feeling great. Her daughter will soon be graduating from law school and getting married, and her son is now in eleventh grade and looking forward to going to college to study engineering. She is presently the medical director for RECNAC II and has dedicated herself to assisting cancer patients in their journey. From her personal experience, she lets them know that there is hope and that cancer is not the death sentence they have been led to believe.

PROSTATE CANCER

E.Z., 57, is a school teacher who was diagnosed with prostate cancer in 2003. He had no history of previous illness. Upon diagnosis, he was started on Lupron (an anti-hormonal drug) every three months and subsequently his condition was apparently stable. In December 2007, a workup was performed due to persistent bone pain and it revealed bone metastasis, for which he was immediately started on radiation therapy. This proved ineffective, so in February 2008 he was started on chemotherapy along with another twelve sessions of radiation therapy. Once again, he had a poor response. Given the aggressiveness of the condition, he was given another round of chemotherapy in April. E.Z. was on narcotic painkillers, anti-emetics, and Lupron every three months, but his health continued deteriorating.

In June, the pain and weakness were so severe, along with his loss of appetite and recurrent insomnia, that he was recommended another round of radiation. He then decided to try the RECNAC II protocol as an attempt to improve his quality of life. In July, he was brought to the office assisted by his family—given the pain he was in, he was unable to walk on his own. E.Z. was started on intravenous vitamin C, oral supplementation, and diet modifications, and by the second dose of the vitamin, he had discontinued the painkillers. Presently, he is sleeping and eating very well, able to walk by himself, performing his basic needs on his own, and showing great improvement in skin color and texture. He feels relaxed and content and is getting his life back.

TESTICULAR CANCER

M.M. is an actor, singer, and graduate psychology student. In 2003, at the age of 29, he started having genitourinary problems: recurrent infections and a mass in one testicle. He was told it was a benign, but the infections continued and he developed abdominal and back pains. The testicle mass continued growing and he was eventually found to have testicular cancer with metastasis to the abdomen and lungs. He underwent cisplatin-based chemotherapy, which did not control his cancer. M.M. then received more aggressive chemotherapy that decreased his strength and energy level to a point that he could not attend college. In addition, his immune system was debilitated (low white blood cell count) and he had recurrent lung infections.

He then met a very compassionate woman named Eliza, who decided to help him. She discovered the RECNAC II project when her father, a prominent physician, got cancer. Eliza and M.M. visited our office to learn about our research and he decided to use the intravenous vitamin C and oral supplement protocol. When he came to see us, M.M. was so weak that he needed help to walk. After just one treatment, he felt more energized and stronger.

He returned to college, with much improvement in his quality of life. His infections stopped and his white blood cell (WBC) count increased substantially, which allowed for surgical intervention for the primary testicular cancer. At the time of surgery, the testicular mass was very large (the size of a grapefruit). He was found to have a tumor inside another tumor: the outer tumor was slow growing but it had a more aggressive, rapidly growing tumor inside. This situation makes chemotherapy worthless, as his experience demonstrated. The follow-up on his abdominal metastasis revealed encapsulation of the tumors. A few months later, M.M. was starring in a major production of the musical *Fiddler on the Roof.* He is currently doing well and advancing in his psychology career as well.

PANCREATIC CANCER

In May 2006, N.D., 70, a nurse, was evaluated for gastrointestinal problems when her physician found that a cancer marker blood test (CEA) had an abnormally high value. Subsequently, a pelvic sonogram revealed a mass in her pancreas. She was diagnosed with pancreatic cancer and given six months to live. Knowing the grim prognosis of her disease even with the most aggressive oncology treatments, she refused conventional therapy in order to preserve the best quality of life for her remaining time.

In June, she started intravenous vitamin C and supplementation along with a vegetarian diet as her sole therapy. This gave her a feeling of renewed vigor and energy. In February 2007, an abdominal sonogram found no abnormal findings and she is now cancer free and doing well.

HODGKIN'S LYMPHOMA (LYMPHATIC CANCER)

D.S. is a young single parent of a four-year-old girl. In January 2006, at the age of 26, she was diagnosed with herpes. Despite receiving medication, she had exacerbations of her viral disease with each menstrual period. With time, she developed a painless enlargement of one lymph node in her neck. In September, she had a biopsy and the pathologist indicated that the cells came from a Hodgkin's lymphoma. A second biopsy from an axillary lymph node, performed in November, confirmed the diagnosis. She started chemotherapy (Dacarbazine, Vinblastine, Bleomycin, and Adriamycin) immediately and received treatment every two weeks.

D.S. was concerned about the toxicity of chemotherapy, so she started looking for professional advice on dietary supplementation to get protection prior to starting treatment. However, she had received two cycles before she found us. By this time, she had already suffered substantial adverse effects—weakness, malaise, upset stomach, depression, insomnia, and dizziness. Her financial situation was tight and she therefore could not stop working in order to regain her health.

She was aware that there is a relationship between viral illnesses and lymphoma and therefore was interested in intravenous vitamin C for both its antiviral effects and its anti-cancer effects. D.S. started the diet and oral and intravenous supplement protocol and her strength and energy levels increased, while her adverse effects decreased. She could eat better, maintain weight, and she felt stronger. She continued working for most of her treatment and felt renewed enthusiasm for life.

Her chemotherapy treatment was completed in April 2007 and she continued oral supplementation. She later received radiotherapy, but unlike most patients who undergo radiotherapy, her skin did not burn or hurt, she never lost her hair (although it got thinner), and her libido was not affected. A follow-up PET scan demonstrated a substantial reduction of the original mass and, better yet, it had no metabolic activity, which meant that the mass was dead tissue. Subsequent imaging revealed continued shrinkage of the mass. She is currently doing well and her viral condition has improved substantially.

E.G., 26, is an accountant and merchandise promoter. In September 2007, while participating in a bodybuilding and physical conditioning program at a local gym, he sensed a swelling in his neck, mainly on the right side. His physician treated it with anti-inflammatory medication and analgesics, but shortly afterward a mass was observed in the region. A biopsy revealed Hodgkin's lymphoma. A PET scan showed neck masses and multiple chest masses.

E.G. was resistant to receiving chemotherapy and decided to start with intravenous vitamin C, oral supplementation, as well as diet and lifestyle modification. In October, after his mother insisting that he use chemotherapy, he was started on Dacarbazine, Vinblastine, Bleomycin, and Adriamycin. But he experienced no hair loss, no weight loss, and continued working regularly; he only experienced an upset stomach and bitter taste in his mouth the day after chemotherapy.

In January 2008, a PET scan showed that his previous neck and chest masses had no metabolic activity. He refused to receive any additional chemotherapy or radiation. He continues sporadically receiving intravenous vitamin C and oral supplements. He has since started his own business and is doing very well. It is gratifying to see how happy he looks, considering that he earlier felt that, with the diagnosis of Hodgkin's lymphoma, his life had come to an end. One of his major fears was that chemotherapy would damage all his systems and that he would never recuperate. After having chemotherapy together with vitamin C and the supplementation protocol, and exhibiting minimal secondary effects, he had the best of both worlds.

Conclusion

"First a new theory is attacked as absurd;
then it is admitted to be true, but obvious and insignificant;
finally, it is seen to be so important that its adversaries
claim they themselves discovered it."
—WILLIAM JAMES (1842–1910)

Although they are slowly changing, oncologists tend to limit or prohibit dietary supplementation. What then happens is that the patient, trusting the clinician, is either denied the benefit of supplementation or conceals supplement use from the doctor.

We appreciate that clinicians are in a tough situation. They are not taught about nutritional supplementation in medical school or during their subsequent specialty training. Continuing medical education and the most prestigious medical journals generally do not cover this area because they are mostly sponsored by pharmaceutical companies that need to promote their products. Occasionally some studies dealing with dietary supplements reach medical journals, and when they do, it is not uncommon that they have methodological problems. We have seen studies selecting the wrong form of a nutrient, incorrect route of administration, wrong dose (very common), or patient population with the wrong severity of disease.

The United States practices a defensive kind of medicine and the system does not facilitate that these nontoxic supplements become part of standard medical treatment guidelines. That is why advancement in this area will be slow.

There are many ways that cancer patients can benefit from the ortho-molecular approach as described in this book. Those benefits are demonstrated by both improved length of life and improved quality of life. Malnourished patients have neither. The combination of conventional and orthomolecular therapy can be of great benefit for patients with early-stage or advanced cancers. Therapy with diet, oral supplementation, or oral and intravenous nutrient protocols can all provide tremendous help when used solely or combined.

We believe that respect for the patient's beliefs and value systems is more important than anything else. That is why some people are willing to give their life for what they believe or for whom they love. It so often doesn't matter what doctors think is best for the patient. Removing a breast cannot be undone; you can reconstruct it, but the physical and emotional pain can be enormous, and that is the reason that radical decisions such as this must not be taken without respecting the patient's values and desires. Refusing to provide a cancer patient with supplemental vitamins and other nutrients is malpractice, and it must stop.

We know that somewhere in heaven Dr. Hugh D. Riordan is smiling with Dr. Linus Pauling, because their dream of providing a better life for cancer patients is becoming a reality.

The time for change has come.

APPENDIX A

Nutritional and Supplemental Protocol

FOOD AS CANCER MEDICINE

Liquids

- Abundance of pure water
- Limited amount of natural juices without added sugar
- No milk; yogurt is okay
- No sodas

Solid Nutrition

- Wholesome and organic grains
- Abundance of multicolored vegetables
- Abundance of sprouted grains
- Fruit—papaya, pineapple, cherry, blueberry, goji, acai berry
- No candy or sugar
- Limited amount of organic low-fat meat
- Fats
  a. No margarine or other partially hydrogenated oils (trans-fatty acids)
  b. No corn oil
  c. Extra-virgin, cold-pressed, organic olive oil
  d. Avocado
  e. Extra-virgin, cold-pressed, organic coconut oil

BIOCHEMICAL OPTIMIZATION, ENERGY FACTORS, AND REPLENISHING FACTORS

Oral Supplementation:

- A high-potency multivitamin/mineral supplement. Take once a day with food.

- Vitamin C. Take 3,000–5,000 mg minimum daily, in divided doses. There is a wide variety of forms of vitamin C. Some, such as the mineral ascorbates, may be more tolerable and are non-acidic. They are also more expensive than regular ascorbic acid.

- Coenzyme Q_{10} (ubiquinol form). Take 100–300 mg daily.

- R-Lipoic acid. Take 300 mg once or twice a day.

- Acetyl L-carnitine. Take 500 mg once or twice a day.

- Omega-3 fish oil (500 mg of EPA, 700 mg of DHA, molecularly distilled). Take 1 capsule, three times a day with meals.

- Iodine. Take 25 mg once a day.

- High-potency digestive enzymes. Take 2–4 tablets, two hours before or after a meal.

- Probiotics (multiple strains formula with 2–4 billion viable organisms and FOS). Take two hours before or after a meal.

- Quercetin. Take 200–400 mg daily.

- Vitamin D. Take 5,000 IU daily.

- Selenium. Take 200 mcg daily.

- Green tea. Take as desired.

NONTOXIC CHEMOTHERAPY

Consider high-dose intravenous vitamin C. If your health-care provider needs information about the application of high-dose intravenous vitamin C, please refer to the following publication: Riordan, H.D., R.B. Hunninghake, N.H. Riordan, et al. "Intravenous Ascorbic Acid: Protocol for Its Application and Use." *P R Health Sci J* 22:2 (2003): 225–232.

Resources on the Nutritional Treatment of Cancer

INTERNET RESOURCES

More on the nutritional treatment of cancer

http://www.doctoryourself.com/cancer.html
http://www.doctoryourself.com/cancer_2.html
http://www.doctoryourself.com/hoffer_vitc_can.html

Dr. Abram Hoffer's comments on nutritional cancer therapy

http://www.doctoryourself.com/cancer_hoffer.html
http://www.doctoryourself.com/hoffer_cancer_2.html
http://www.doctoryourself.com/hoffer_niacin.html

Dr. Hugh Riordan's use of vitamin C as chemotherapy

http://www.doctoryourself.com/riordan2.html
http://www.doctoryourself.com/riordan1.html
http://www.doctoryourself.com/biblio_riordan.html

Dr. Ewan Cameron's vitamin C protocol for cancer patients

http://www.doctoryourself.com/cameron.html

Why vitamin C does not interfere with drug chemotherapy

http://www.doctoryourself.com/chemo.html

The Gerson cancer therapy

http://www.doctoryourself.com/gersontherapy.html
http://www.doctoryourself.com/gersonbio.htm
http://www.doctoryourself.com/gersonspeech.html
http://www.doctoryourself.com/bib_gerson.html
http://www.doctoryourself.com/bib_gerson_therapy.html

SELECTED LIST OF LINUS PAULING'S PAPERS ON VITAMIN C AND CANCER

Pauling, L. "Supplemental Ascorbate in the Supportive Treatment of Cancer: Prolongation of Survival Times in Terminal Human Cancer." *Proc Natl Acad Sci U S A* 73 (1976): 3685–3689.

Pauling, L. "Ascorbic Acid and Cancer." *Natl Acad Prev Med J* 1 (1976): 6–10.

Pauling, L. "Diet, Nutrition, and Cancer." *Am J Clin Nutr* 30 (1977): 661, 663.

Pauling, L. "Vitamin C and Cancer." *Linus Pauling Inst Sci Med Newsletter* 1:2 (1977): 1–2.

Cameron, E., and L. Pauling. "Vitamin C and Cancer." *Intl J Environ Studies* 10 (1977), 303–305.

Pauling, L. "Supplemental Ascorbate in the Supportive Treatment of Cancer: Prolongation of Survival Times in Terminal Human Cancer." *J Natural Med* 1:2 (May/June 1977).

Cameron, E., and L. Pauling. "Supplemental Ascorbate in the Supportive Treatment of Cancer: Reevaluation of Prolongation of Survival Times in Terminal Human Cancer." *Proc Natl Acad Sci U S A* 75 (1978): 4538–4542.

Cameron, E., and L. Pauling. "Experimental Studies Designed to Evaluate the Management of Patients with Incurable Cancer." *Proc Natl Acad Sci U S A* 75 (1978): 6252.

Cameron, E., and L. Pauling. "Ascorbic Acid as a Therapeutic Agent in Cancer." *J Intl Acad Prev Med* 5:1 (1978): 8–29.

Cameron, E., L. Pauling, B. Leibovitz. "Ascorbic Acid and Cancer: A Review." *Cancer Res* 39 (1979): 663–681.

Pauling, L. "Ascorbic Acid." *Lancet* 1 (1979): 615.

Cameron, E., and L. Pauling. "Ascorbate and Cancer." *Proc Am Phil Soc* 123 (1979): 117–123.

Pauling, L. "The Role of Vitamin C in Cancer." *Intl J Vitamin Nutr Res Suppl* 19 (1979): 207–210.

Pauling, L. "Ascorbic Acid as a Therapeutic Agent in Cancer." *J Intl Acad Prev Med* V:1 (1979): 8–29.

Pauling, L. "Vitamin C Therapy of Advanced Cancer." *New Engl J Med* 302 (1980): 694–695.

Cameron, E., and L. Pauling. "Survival Times of Terminal Lung Cancer Patients Treated with Ascorbate." *J Intl Acad Prev Med* 6 (1981): 21–27.

Dunham, W.B., E. Zuckerkandl, R. Reynolds, et al. "Effects of Intake of L-Ascorbic Acid on the Incidence of Dermal Neoplasms Induced in Mice by Ultraviolet Light." *Proc Natl Acad Sci U S A* 79 (1982): 7532–7536.

Pauling, L., R. Willoughby, R. Reynolds, et al. "Incidence of Squamous Cell Carcinoma in Hairless Mice Irradiated with Ultraviolet Light in Relation to Intake of Ascorbic Acid (Vitamin C) and of D,L-Alpha-tocopheryl Acetate (Vitamin E)." In Hanck, A. (ed.). *Vitamin C: New Clinical Applications in Immunology, Lipid Metabolism, and Cancer.* (*Intl J Vitamin Nutr Res* Suppl 23.) Bern: Hans Huber Publishers, 1982, 53–82.

Kimoto, E., H. Tanaka, J. Gyotoku, et al. "Enhancement of Antitumor Activity of Ascorbate against Ehrlich Ascites Tumor Cells by the Copper:glycylglycylhistidine Complex." *Cancer Res* 43 (1983): 824–828.

Cameron, E., and L. Pauling. "Vitamin C and Cancer." *Australas Health Healing* 2:3 (April–June 1983): 9–10.

APPENDIX C

RECNAC II Publications

Casciari, J.J., H.D. Riordan, J.R. Miranda-Massari, et al. "Effects of High-dose Ascorbate Administration on L-10 Tumor Growth in Guinea Pigs." *P R Health Sci* J 24 (2005): 145–150.

Duconge, J., J.R. Miranda-Massari, M.J. González, et al. "Pharmacokinetics of Vitamin C: Insights into the Oral and Intravenous Administration of Ascorbate." *P R Health Sci J* 27 (February 2008): 7–19.

Duconge, J., J.R. Miranda-Massari, M.J. González, et al. "Vitamin C Pharmacokinetics after Continuous Intravenous Infusion in a Prostate Cancer Patient." *Ann Pharmacother* 41:6 (2007): 1082–1083.

Duconge, J., J.R. Miranda-Massari, M.J. González, et al. "Schedule-dependence in Cancer Therapy: What is the True Scenario for Vitamin C?" *J Orthomolecular Med* 22 (2007): 21–26.

González, M.J., and J.R. Miranda-Massari. "Advances in Vitamin C Research." *Integr Cancer Ther* 5 (2006): 7–8.

González, M.J., J.R. Miranda-Massari, H.D. Riordan. "Vitamin C as an Ergogenic Aid." *J Orthomolecular Med* 20 (2005): 23–27.

González, M.J., J.R. Miranda-Massari, et al. "Nutritional Oncology Review: Ascorbic Acid and Cancer: 25 Years Later." *Integr Cancer Ther* 4 (2005): 32–44.

González, M.J., J.R. Miranda-Massari, H.D. Riordan. "The Vitamin C and DNA Damage Revisited." *J Orthomolecular Med* 17 (2002): 225–228.

González, M.J., E.M. Mora, J.R. Miranda-Massari, et al. "Inhibition of Human Breast Carcinoma Cell Proliferation by Ascorbate and Copper." *P R Health Sci J* 21 (2002): 21–23.

González, M.J., E.M. Mora, J.R. Miranda-Massari, et al. "Orthomolecular Oncology: A Mechanistic View of Intravenous Ascorbate Chemotherapeutic Activity." *P R Health Sci J* 21 (2002): 39–41.

González, M.J., J.R. Miranda-Massari, A. Guzmán, et al. "Non-Toxic

Chemotherapy for Cancer." (Abstract.) First Inter-American Conference of Pharmacy and Nutrition, Havana, Cuba, June 2001.

González, M.J., M.I. Matos, J.R. Miranda-Massari, et al. "Integrative Medicine, an Innovative Approach to Medical Education and Practice." *P R Health Sci J* 19:4 (2000): 389–392.

Kumar, S., J.R. Miranda-Massari, M.J. González, et al. "Intravenous Ascorbic Acid as a Treatment for Severe Jellyfish Stings." *P R Health Sci J* 23 (2004): 125–126.

Meng, X.L., N.H. Riordan, H.D. Riordan, et al. "Fatty Acid Composition Variability between Normal and Malignant Cell Lines." *P R Health Sci J* 23 (2004): 103–106.

Meng, X.L., N.H. Riordan, J.J. Casciari, et al. "Effects of a High Molecular Mass *Convolvus arvensis* Extract on Tumor Growth and Angiogenesis." *P R Health Sci J* 21:4 (2002): 323–328.

Mikirova, N.A., H.D. Riordan, J.A. Jackson, et al. "Erythrocyte Membrane Fatty Acid Composition in Cancer Patients." *P R Health Sci J* 23 (2004): 107–114.

Miranda-Massari, J.R., and M.J. González. "Toward a New Era in Research, Education and Healing." (Editorial Comment.) *P R Health Sci J* 23 (2004): 85–86.

Miranda-Massari, J.R., and M.J. González. "Integrative Medicine: An Innovative Approach to Medicine and Medical Education for the Next Millennium." *Biomedicina* 3:1 (2000): s5–s6.

Pérez, Y., A. Guzmán, E. Mora, et al. "Ascorbic Acid and Copper: Effective Cytoxic Agents Against Metastatic Breast Carcinoma (*BRCA*) Cells." (Poster 1150.) *Proc Am Assoc Cancer Res* (ACCR) (March 2001): 42.

Riordan, H.D., J.J. Casciari, M.J. González, et al. "A Pilot Clinical Study of Continuous Intravenous Ascorbate in Terminal Cancer Patients." *P R Health Sci J* 24 (2005): 269–276.

Riordan, H.D., N.H. Riordan, J.A. Jackson, et al. "Intravenous Vitamin C as a Chemotherapy Agent: A Report on Clinical Cases." *P R Health Sci J* 23 (2004): 115–118.

Riordan, H.D., R.B. Hunninghake, N.H. Riordan, et al. "Intravenous Ascorbic Acid: Protocol for Its Application and Use." *P R Health Sci J* 22:2 (2003): 225–232.

Rosario-Pérez, G., M.J. González, A.M. Guzmán, et al. "Ascorbic Acid, Mitochondria and Cancer." *Revista Puertorriqueña de Medicina y Salud Pública* 14 (2009): 103–108.

References

Chapter 1: Not a Death Sentence

1. Riordan, H.D. *Medical Mavericks, Vol. I.* Wichita, KS: Bio-Communications Press, 1988. Riordan, H.D. *Medical Mavericks, Vol. II.* Wichita, KS: Bio-Communications Press, 1989. Riordan, H.D. *Medical Mavericks, Vol. III.* Wichita, KS: Bio-Communications Press, 2005.

2. Levine, M., K.R. Dhariwal, P. Washko, et al. "Ascorbic Acid and Reaction Kinetics in situ: A New Approach to Vitamin Requirements." *J Nutr Sci Vitaminol* (Tokyo) (1992): 169–172. Wang, Y.H., K.R. Dhariwal, M. Levine. "Ascorbic Acid Bioavailability in Humans. Ascorbic Acid in Plasma, Serum, and Urine." *Ann N Y Acad Sci* 669 (September 1992): 383–386. Padayatty, S.J., H. Sun, Y. Wang, et al. "Vitamin C Pharmacokinetics: Implications for Oral and Intravenous Use." *Ann Intern Med* 140:7 (April 2004): 533–537. Chen, Q., M.G. Espey, M.C. Krishna, et al. "Pharmacologic Ascorbic Acid Concentrations Selectively Kill Cancer Cells: Action as a Pro-drug to Deliver Hydrogen Peroxide to Tissues." *Proc Natl Acad Sci U S A* 102:38 (September 2005): 13604–13609.

3. Cameron, E., L. Pauling, B. Leibovitz. "Ascorbic Acid and Cancer: A Review." *Cancer Res* 39 (1979): 663–681.

Chapter 2: Knowing the Enemy

1. Gonzalez, M.J., E.M. Mora, J.R. Miranda-Massari, et al. "Inhibition of Human Breast Carcinoma Cell Proliferation by Ascorbate and Copper." *P R Health Sci J* 21:1 (March 2002): 21–23.

2. Chen, Q., M.G. Espey, M.C. Krishna, et al. "Pharmacologic Ascorbic Acid Concentrations Selectively Kill Cancer Cells: Action as a Pro-drug to Deliver Hydrogen Peroxide to Tissues." *Proc Natl Acad Sci U S A* 102:38 (September 2005): 13604–13609.

3. Riordan, H.D., J.J. Casciari, M.J. Gonzalez, et al. "A Pilot Clinical Study of Continuous Intravenous Ascorbate in Terminal Cancer Patients." *P R Health Sci J* 24:4 (December 2005): 269–276.

4. Chen, Q., M.G. Espey, M.C. Krishna, et al. "Pharmacologic Ascorbic Acid Concentrations Selectively Kill Cancer Cells: Action as a Pro-drug to Deliver Hydrogen Peroxide to Tissues." *Proc Natl Acad Sci U S A* 102:38 (September 2005): 13604–13609.

5. Cameron, E., and L. Pauling. "Supplemental Ascorbate in the Supportive Treatment of Cancer: Prolongation of Survival Times in Terminal Human Cancer." *Proc Natl Acad Sci U S A* 73:10 (October 1976): 3685–3689. Creagan, E.T., C.G. Moertel, J.R. O'Fallon, et al. "Failure of High-dose Vitamin C (Ascorbic Acid) Therapy to Benefit Patients with Advanced Cancer. A Controlled Trial." *N Engl J Med* 301:13 (September 1979): 687–690.

6. Chen, Q., M.G. Espey, A.Y. Sun, et al. "Pharmacologic Doses of Ascorbate Act as a Prooxidant and Decrease Growth of Aggressive Tumor Xenografts in Mice." *Proc Natl Acad Sci U S A* 105:32 (2008): 11105–11109.

7. Agus, D.B., J.C. Vera, D.W. Golde. "Stromal Cell Oxidation: A Mechanism by which Tumors Obtain Vitamin C." *Cancer Res* 59 (1999): 4555–4558.

8. Casciari, J.J., H.D. Riordan, J.R. Miranda-Massari, et al. "Effects of High-dose Ascorbate Administration on L-10 Tumor Growth in Guinea Pigs." *P R Health Sci J* 24 (2005): 145–150.

9. Riordan, H.D., J.J. Casciari, M.J. González, et al. "A Pilot Clinical Study of Continuous Intravenous Ascorbate in Terminal Cancer Patients." *P R Health Sci J* 24 (2005): 269–276.

10. Morgan, G., R. Ward, M. Barton. "The Contribution of Cytotoxic Chemotherapy to 5-year Survival in Adult Malignancies." *Clin Oncol (R Coll Radiol)* 16:8 (December 2004): 549–560.

Chapter 3: Food as Cancer Medicine

1. King, W.D., and L.D. Marrett. "Case-control Study of Bladder Cancer and Chlorination By-products in Treated Water (Ontario, Canada)." *Cancer Causes Control* 7:6 (November 1996): 596–604. Anonymous. "NIEHS News. Trihalomethanes and Colorectal Cancer." *Environ Health Perspect* 102:2 (February 1994): 151–152. Morris, R.D. "Environmental Health Issues: Drinking Water and Cancer." *Environ Health Perspect* 103:Suppl 8 (November 1995): 225–231. Kasim, K., P. Levallois, K.C. Johnson, et al., and the Canadian Cancer Registries Epidemiology Research Group. "Chlorination Disinfection By-products in Drinking Water and the Risk of Adult Leukemia in Canada." *Am J Epidemiol* 163:2 (January 2006): 116–126.

2. Cedergrena, M.I., A.J. Selbinga, O. Löfmanb, et al. "Chlorination Byproducts and Nitrate in Drinking Water and Risk for Congenital Cardiac Defects." *Environ Res* 89:2 (June 2002): 124–130. Hwang, B-F., P. Magnus, J.J.K. Jaakkola. "Risk of Specific Birth Defects in Relation to Chlorination and the Amount

of Natural Organic Matter in the Water Supply." *Am J Epidemiol* 156:4 (August 2002): 374–382.

3. Magnus, P., J.J.K. Jaakkola, A. Skrondal;, et al. "Water Chlorination and Birth Defects." *Epidemiology* 10:5 (September 1999): 513–517.

4. Waller, K., S.H. Swan, G. DeLorenze et al. "Trihalomethanes in Drinking Water and Spontaneous Abortion." *Epidemiology* 9:2 (March 1998): 134–140.

5. Villanueva, C.M., K.P. Cantor, J.O. Grimalt, et al. "Bladder Cancer and Exposure to Water Disinfection By-Products through Ingestion, Bathing, Showering, and Swimming in Pools." *Am J Epidemiol* 165:2 (January 2007): 148–156.

6. Patterson, B.H., G. Block, W.F. Rosenberger, et al. "Fruit and Vegetables in the American Diet: Data from the NHANES II Survey." *Am J Public Health* 80:12 (December 1990): 1443–1449.

7. Foster, H.D. *Reducing Cancer Mortality: A Geographical Perspective.* Western Geographical Series, Vol. 23. Victoria, Canada: Western Geographical Press, 1986.

8. Slavin, J. "Whole Grains and Human Health." *Nutr Res Rev* 17 (2004): 99–110.

9. Linos, E., W.C. Willett, E. Cho, et al. "Red Meat Consumption during Adolescence among Premenopausal Women and Risk of Breast Cancer." *Cancer Epidemiol Biomarkers Prev* 17:8 (August 2008): 2146–2151.

10. Gonzalez, M.J. "Fish Oil, Lipid Peroxidation and Mammary Tumor Growth." *J Am Coll Nutr* 14:4 (1995): 325–335. Kato, T., N. Kolenic, R.S. Pardini. "Docosahexaenoic Acid (DHA), a Primary Tumor Suppressive Omega-3 Fatty Acid, Inhibits Growth of Colorectal Cancer Independent of *p53* Mutational Status." *Nutr Cancer* 58:2 (2007): 178–187. Yin, Y., W.H. Zhan, J.S. Peng, et al. ["Apoptosis of Human Gastric Cancer Cells Induced by Omega-3 Polyunsaturated Fatty Acids."] *Zhonghua Wei Chang Wai Ke Za Zhi* 10:6 (November 2007): 570–573. Zhang, W., Y. Long, J. Zhang, et al. "Modulatory Effects of EPA and DHA on Proliferation and Apoptosis of Pancreatic Cancer Cells." *J Huazhong Univ Sci Technolog Med Sci* 27:5 (October 2007): 547–550.

11. Tapiero, H., G.N. Ba, P. Couvreur, et al. "Polyunsaturated Fatty Acids (PUFA) and Eicosanoids in Human Health and Pathologies." *Biomed Pharmacother* 56:5 (July 2002): 215–222.

12. Das, U.N. "Essential Fatty Acids: Biochemistry, Physiology and Pathology." *Biotechnol J* 1:4 (April 2006): 420–439.

13. Kundu, J.K., and Y.J. Surh. "Inflammation: Gearing the Journey to Cancer." *Mutat Res* 659:1–2 (July–August 2008): 15–30.

14. Chen, J., K.A. Power, J. Mann, et al. "Flaxseed Alone or in Combination with

Tamoxifen Inhibits MCF-7 Breast Tumor Growth in Ovariectomized Athymic Mice with High Circulating Levels of Estogen." *Exp Biol Med (Maywood)* 232:8 (September 2007): 1071–1080.

15. Waite, N., J. Lodge, K. Hart, et al. "The Impact of Fish-Oil Supplements on Insulin Sensitivity." *J Hum Nutr Diet* 21:4 (July 2008): 402–403.

16. Kromhout, D., E.B. Bosschieter, C. de Lezenne Coulander. "The Inverse Relation between Fish Consumption and 20-Year Mortality from Coronary Heart Disease." *New Engl J Med* 312 (1985): 1205.

17. Hoehn, S.K., et al. "Complex versus Simple Carbohydrates and Mammary Tumors in Mice." *Nutr Cancer* 1:3 (1979): 27.

18. Sanchez, A., J.L. Reeser, H.S. Lau, et al. "Role of Sugars in Human Neutrophilic Phagocytosis." *Am J Clin Nutr* 26:11 (1973): 1180–1184.

19. Santisteban, G.A., J.T. Ely, E.E. Hamel, et al. "Glycemic Modulation of Tumor Tolerance in a Mouse Model of Breast Cancer." *Biochem Biophys Res Commun* 132:3 (1985): 1174–1179.

20. Seeley, S. "Diet and Breast Cancer: The Possible Connection with Sugar Consumption." *Med Hypotheses* 11 (1983): 319–327.

21. For more about Gerson Therapy: Gerson, C., and B. Bishop. *Healing the Gerson Way*. Carmel, CA: Totality Books, 2007. Gerson, Charlotte, and Morton Walker, DPM. *The Gerson Therapy*. New York: Kensington Publishing, 2001. For a transcript of a speech by Dr. Gerson, see http://www.doctoryourself.com/ gerson speech.html. A bibliography of published clinical studies showing the benefits of the Gerson treatment is available online at http://www.doctoryourself.com/ bib_gerson_therapy.html. A complete bibliography of Dr. Gerson's scientific writings is available at http://www.doctoryourself.com/bib_gerson.html.

22. Bounous, G. "Whey Protein Concentrate (WPC) and Glutathione Modulation in Cancer Treatment." *Anticancer Res* 20:6C (November-December 2000): 4785–4792.

23. Ames, B.N. "The Metabolic Tune-Up: Metabolic Harmony and Disease Prevention." *J Nutr* 133 (2003): 1544S–1548S.

24. Bowen, P., L. Chen, M. Stacewicz-Sapuntzakis, et al. "Tomato Sauce Supplementation and Prostate Cancer: Lycopene Accumulation and Modulation of Biomarkers of Carcinogenesis." *Exp Biol Med* 227:10 (November 2002): 886–893.

25. Rao, A.V., and S. Agarwal. "Role of Antioxidant Lycopene in Cancer and Heart Disease." *J Am Coll Nutr* 19:5 (October 2000): 563–569.

Chapter 4: Biochemical Optimization for Cancer Patients

1. Reginster, J.Y., R. Deroisy, L.C. Rovati, et al. "Long-term Effects of Glucosamine Sulphate on Osteoarthritis Progression: A Randomised, Placebo-

controlled Clinical Trial." *Lancet* 357:9252 (2001): 251–256. Pavelka, K., J. Gatterova, M. Olejarova, et al. "Glucosamine Sulfate Use and Delay of Progression of Knee Osteoarthritis: A 3-year, Randomized, Placebo-controlled, Double-blind Study." *Arch Intern Med* 162:18 (2002): 2113–2123. Buyere, O., K. Pavelka, L.C. Rovati, et al. "Glucosamine Sulfate Reduces Osteoarthritis Progression in Postmenopausal Women with Knee Osteoarthritis: Evidence from Two 3-year Studies." *Menopause* 11:2 (2004): 138–143. Buyere, O., K. Pavelka, L.C. Rovati, et al. "Total Joint Replacement after Glucosamine Sulphate Treatment in Knee Osteoarthritis: Results of a Mean 8-year Observation of Patients from Two Previous 3-year, Randomised, Placebo-controlled Trials." *Osteoarth Cartilage* 16:2 (2008): 254–260.

2. Williams, Roger. *The Wonderful World Within You: Your Inner Nutritional Environment.* New York: Bantam Books, 1977.

3. Ames, B.N. "A Role for Supplements in Optimizing Health: The Metabolic Tune-up." *Arch Biochem Biophys* 423:1 (March 2004): 227–234.

4. Ames, B.N., H. Atamna, D.W. Killilea. "Mineral and Vitamin Deficiencies Can Accelerate the Mitochondrial Decay of Aging." *Mol Aspects Med* 26:4–5 (August-October 2005): 363–378.

5. Jager, R., J. Metzger, K. Lautmann, et al. "The Effects of Creatine Pyruvate and Creatine Citrate on Performance during High-intensity Exercise." *J Intl Soc Sports Nutr* 5 (February 2008): 4. Dragan, G.I., E. Ploesteanu, V. Selejan. "Studies Concerning the Ergogenic Value of Cantamega-2000 Supply in Top Junior Cyclists." *Rev Roum Physiol* 28:1–2 (1991): 13–16. Cramer, J.T., J.R. Stout, J.Y. Culbertson, et al. "Effects of Creatine Supplementation and Three Days of Resistance Training on Muscle Strength, Power Output, and Neuromuscular Function." *J Strength Cond Res* 21:3 (August 2007): 668–677.

6. Schmier, J.K., N.J. Rachman, M.T. Halpern. "The Cost-effectiveness of Omega-3 Supplements for Prevention of Secondary Coronary Events." *Manag Care* 15:4 (April 2006): 43–50.

7. Gariballa, S., and S. Forster. "Dietary Supplementation and Quality of Life of Older Patients: A Randomized, Double-blind, Placebo-controlled Trial." *J Am Geriatr Soc* 55:12 (December 2007): 2030–2034.

8. Misnerm, B. "Food Alone May Not Provide Sufficient Micronutrients for Preventing Deficiency." *J Intl Soc Sports Nutr* 3:1 (2006): 51–55.

9. American Dietetic Association. "Position of the American Dietetic Association: Fortification and Nutritional Supplements." *J Am Diet Assoc* 105:8 (August 2005): 1300–1311. Fairfield, K.M., and R.H. Fletcher. "Vitamins for Chronic Disease Prevention in Adults: Scientific Review." *JAMA* 287 (2002): 3116–3126. Fletcher, R.H., and K.M. Fairfield. "Vitamins for Chronic Disease Prevention in Adults: Clinical Applications." *JAMA* 287 (2002): 3127–3129.

10. Gloth III, F.M., J. Tobin, C. Smith, et al. "Nutrient Intakes in a Frail Home-bound Elderly Population in the Community vs. a Nursing Home Population." *J Am Diet Assoc* 96:6 (1996): 605–607.

11. Sebastian, R.S., L.E. Cleveland, J.D. Goldman, et al. "Older Adults Who Use Vitamin/Mineral Supplements Differ from Nonusers in Nutrient Intake Adequacy and Dietary Attitudes." *J Am Diet Assoc* 107:8 (August 2007): 1322–1332.

12. Warburg, O. "On the Origin of Cancer Cells." *Science* 123:3191 (1956): 309–314.

13. van Poppel, G., and H. van den Berg. "Vitamins and Cancer." *Cancer Lett* 114:1–2 (March 1997): 195–202. Arasaradnam, R.P., D.M. Commane, D. Bradburn, et al. "A Review of Dietary Factors and Its Influence on DNA Methylation in Colorectal Carcinogenesis." *Epigenetics* 3 (2008): 193–198.

14. Szyf, M., P. Pakneshan, S.A. Rabbani. "DNA Demethylation and Cancer: Therapeutic Implications." *Cancer Lett* 211:2 (2004): 133–143.

15. Scambia, G., F.O. Raneletti, P.B. Panici, et al. "Quercetin Induces Type-II Estrogen-binding Sites in Estrogen-receptor-negative (MDA-MB231) and Estrogen-receptor-positive (MCF-7) Human Breast-cancer Cell Lines." *Intl J Cancer* 54 (1993): 462–466. Scambia, G., F.O. Raneletti, P.B. Panici, et al. "Quercetin Inhibits the Growth of a Multidrug-resistant Estrogen-receptor-negative MCF-7 Human Breast-cancer Cell Line Expressing Type II Estrogen-binding Sites." *Cancer Chemother Pharmacol* 28 (1991): 255–258. Singhal, R.L., Y.A. Yeh, N. Prajda, et al. "Quercetin Down-regulates Signal Transduction in Human Breast Carcinoma Cells." *Biochem Biophys Res Comm* 208 (1995): 425–431.

16. Larocca, L.M., L. Teofili, S. Sica, et al. "Quercetin Inhibits the Growth of Leukemic Progenitors and Induces the Expression of Transforming Growth Factor-B1 in These Cells." *Blood* 85 (1995): 3654–3661. Larocca, L.M., L. Teofili, G. Leone, et al. "Antiproliferative Activity of Quercetin on Normal Bone Marrow and Leukaemic Progenitors." *Br J Haematol* 79 (1991): 562–566.

17. Pereira, M.A., C.J. Grubbs, L.H. Barnes, et al. "Effects of the Phytochemicals, Curcumin and Quercetin, Upon Azoxymethane-induced Colon Cancer and 7,12-Dimethylbenzy[a]anthracene-induced Mammary Cancer in Rats." *Carcinogenesis* 17 (1996): 1305–1311.

18. Scambia, G., F.O. Raneletti, P.B. Panici, et al. "Inhibitory Effect of Quercetin on Primary Ovarian and Endometrial Cancers and Synergistic Activity with cis-Diamminedichloroplatinum(II)." *Gynecol Oncol* 45 (1992): 13–19. Also: Scambia, G., F.O. Raneletti, P.B. Panici, et al. "Synergistic Antiproliferative Activity of Quercetin and Cisplatin on Ovarian Cancer Cell Growth." *Anticancer Drugs* 1 (1990): 45–48.

19. Yoshida, M., T. Sakai, N. Hosokawa, et al. "The Effect of Quercetin on Cell Cycle Progression and Growth of Human Gastric Cancer Cells." *FEBS Lett* 260 (1990): 10–13.

20. Caltagirone, S., F.O. Raneletti, A. Rinelli, et al. "Interaction with Type II Estrogen Binding Sites and Antiproliferative Activity of Tamoxifen and Quercetin in Human Non-small-cell Lung Cancer." *Am J Resp Cell Mol Biol* 17 (1997): 51–59.

21. Russo, M.W., S.C. Murray , J.I. Wurzelmann, et al. "Plasma Selenium Levels and the Risk of Colorectal Adenomas." *Nutr Cancer* 28 (1997): 125–129. Patterson, B.H., and O.A. Levander. "Naturally Occurring Selenium Compounds in Cancer Chemoprevention Trials: A Workshop Summary." *Cancer Epidemiol Biomarkers Prev* 6 (1997): 63–69. Knekt, P., J. Marniemi, L. Teppo, et al. "Is Low Selenium Status a Risk Factor for Lung Cancer?" *Am J Epidemiol* 148 (1998): 975–982. Fleet, J.C. "Dietary Selenium Repletion May Reduce Cancer Incidence in People at High Risk Who Live in Areas with Low Soil Selenium." *Nutr Rev* 55 (1997): 277–279. Shamberger, R.J. "The Genotoxicity of Selenium." *Mutat Res* 154 (1985): 29–48. Young, K.L., and P.N. Lee. "Intervention Studies on Cancer." *Eur J Cancer Prev* 8 (1999): 91–103.

22. Arbogast, D., G. Bailey, V. Breinholt, et al. "Dietary Chlorophyllin is a Potent Inhibitor of Aflatoxin B1 Hepatocarcinogenesis in Rainbow Trout." *Cancer Res* 55 (1995): 57–62.

23. Sarkar, D., A. Sharma, G. Talukder. "Chlorophyll and Chlorophyllin as Modifiers of Genotoxic Effects." *Mutation Res* 318 (1994): 239–247.

24. Chernomorsky, S., R. Poretz, A. Segelman. "Effect of Dietary Chlorophyll Derivatives on Mutagenesis and Tumor Cell Growth." *Teratogen Carcinogen Mutagen* 79 (1999): 313–322.

25. Lamson, D.W., and S.M. Plaza. "The Anti-cancer Effects of Vitamin K." *Altern Med Rev* 8:3 (August 2003): 303–318.

26. Matzno, S., Y. Yamaguchi, T. Akiyoshi, et al. "An Attempt to Evaluate the Effect of Vitamin K$_3$ Using as an Enhancer of Anti-cancer Agents." *Biol Pharm Bull* 31:6 (2008): 1270–1273.

27. Nishino, H., M. Murakosh, T. Ii, et al. "Carotenoids in Cancer Chemoprevention." *Cancer Metastasis Rev* 21:3–4 (2002): 257–264.

28. Ashrafi, M., S.Z. Bathaie, M. Taghikhani, et al. "The Effect of Carotenoids Obtained from Saffron on Histone H1 Structure and H1-DNA Interaction." *Intl J Biol Macromol* 36:4 (September 2005): 246–252. Nair, S.C., S.K. Kurumboor, J.H. Hasegawa. "Saffron Chemoprevention in Biology and Medicine: A Review." *Cancer Biother* 10:4 (Winter 1995): 257–264.

29. Donato, L.J., J.H. Suh, N. Noy. "Suppression of Mammary Carcinoma Cell

Growth by Retinoic Acid: The Cell Cycle Control Gene *Btg2* is a Direct Target for Retinoic Acid Receptor Signaling." *Cancer Res* 67:2 (January 2007): 609–615.

30. Lopez-Lazaro, M. "Anti-cancer and Carcinogenic Properties of Curcumin: Considerations for Its Clinical Development as a Cancer Chemopreventive and Chemotherapeutic Agent." *Mol Nutr Food Res* 52:Suppl 1 (2008): S103–S127. Mosley, C.A., D.C. Liotta, J.P. Snyder. "Highly Active Anti-cancer Curcumin Analogues." *Adv Exp Med Biol* 595 (2007): 77–103.

31. Aggarwal, B.B., and S. Shishodia. "Molecular Targets of Dietary Agents for Prevention and Therapy of Cancer." *Biochem Pharmacol* 71:10 (May 2006): 1397–1421.

32. Choi, H., Y.S. Chun, S.W. Kim, et al. "Curcumin Inhibits Hypoxia-Inducible Factor-1 by Degrading Aryl Hydrocarbon Receptor Nuclear Translocator: A Mechanism of Tumor Growth Inhibition." *Mol Pharmacol* 70:5 (November 2006): 1664–1671.

33. Herman-Antosiewicz, A., A.A. Powolny, S.V. Singh. "Molecular Targets of Cancer Chemoprevention by Garlic-derived Organosulfides." *Acta Pharmacol Sin* 28:9 (2007): 1355–1364.

34. Seki, T., T. Hosono, T. Hosono-Fukao, et al. "Anti-cancer Effects of Diallyl Trisulfide Derived from Garlic." *Asia Pac J Clin Nutr* 17:Suppl 1 (2008): 249–252.

35. Dulloo, A.G., C. Duret, D. Rohrer, et al. "Efficacy of a Green Tea Extract Rich in Catechin Polyphenols and Caffeine in Increasing 24-h Energy Expenditure and Fat Oxidation in Humans." *Am J Clin Nutr* 70 (1999): 1040–1045.

36. Mittal, A., M. Pate, R. Wylie, et al. "EGCG Down-regulates Telomerase in Human Breast Carcinoma MCF-7 Cells, Leading to Suppression of Cell Viability and Induction of Apoptosis." *Intl J Oncol* 24 (2004): 703–710. Khan, N., and H. Mukhtar. "Multitargeted Therapy of Cancer by Green Tea Polyphenols." *Cancer Lett* 269:2 (2008): 269–280.

37. Sartippour, M.R., Z.M. Shao, D. Heber, et al. "Green Tea Inhibits Vascular Endothelial Growth Factor (VEGF) Induction in Human Breast Cancer Cells." *J Nutr* 132 (2002): 2307–2311.

38. Heilbrun, L.K., A. Nomura, G.N. Stemmermann. "Black Tea Consumption and Cancer Risk: A Prospective Study." *Br J Cancer* 54 (1986): 677–683. Also: Jain, M.G., G.T. Hislop, G.R. Howe, et al. "Alcohol and Other Beverage Use and Prostate Cancer Risk among Canadian Men." *Intl J Cancer* 78:6 (1998): 707–711. Jian, L., L.L.P. Xie, A.H. Lee, et al. "Protective Effect of Green Tea against Prostate Cancer: A Case-control Study in Southeast China." *Intl J Cancer* 108 (2004): 130–135.

39. Bettuzzi, S., M. Brausi, F. Rizzi, et al. "Chemoprevention of Human Prostate Cancer by Oral Administration of Green Tea Catechins in Volunteers with High-grade Prostate Intraepithelial Neoplasia: A Preliminary Report from a One-year Proof-of-principle Study." *Cancer Res* 66 (2006): 1234–1240. Imai, K., K. Suga, K. Nakachi. "Cancer Preventing Effects of Drinking Green Tea among Japanese Population." *Prev Med* 26 (1997): 769–775.

40. Chen, Q., M.G. Espey, M.C. Krishna, et al. "Pharmacologic Ascorbic Acid Concentrations Selectively Kill Cancer Cells: Action as a Pro-drug to Deliver Hydrogen Peroxide to Tissues." *Proc Natl Acad Sci U S A* 102:38 (2005): 13604–13609.

41. Stoll, K.E., and J.R. Duncan. "The Effect of Ascorbic Acid on Arachidonic Acid and Prostaglandin E2 Metabolism in B16 Murine Melanoma Cells." *Prostaglandins Leukot Essent Fatty Acids* 47:4 (December 1992): 307–312.

42. Chen, Q., M.G. Espey, M.C. Krishna, et al. "Pharmacologic Ascorbic Acid Concentrations Selectively Kill Cancer Cells: Action as a Pro-drug to Deliver Hydrogen Peroxide to Tissues." *Proc Natl Acad Sci U S A* 102:38 (2005): 13604–13609.

43. Klenner, F.R. "The Treatment of Poliomyelitis and Other Virus Diseases with Vitamin C." *South Med Surg* 3 (1949): 7–12.

44. McCormick, W.J. "Ascorbic Acid as Chemotherapeutic Agent." *Arch Pediatr* 69 (1952): 151–155.

45. Padayatty, S.J., A. Katz, Y. Wang, et al. "Vitamin C as an Antioxidant: Evaluation of Its Role in Disease Prevention." *J Am Coll Nutr* 22:1 (2003): 18–35. Gonzalez, M.J., J.R. Miranda-Massari, E.M. Mora, et al. "Orthomolecular Oncology Review: Ascorbic Acid and Cancer 25 Years Later." *Integr Cancer Ther* 4:1 (2005): 32–44.

46. Hercberg, S., P. Galan, P. Preziosi, et al. "The SU.VI.MAX Study: A Randomized, Placebo-controlled Trial of the Health Effects of Antioxidant Vitamins and Minerals." *Arch Intern Med* 164:21 (2004): 2335–2342.

47. Meyer, F., P. Galan, P. Douville, et al. "Antioxidant Vitamin and Mineral Supplementation and Prostate Cancer Prevention in the SU.VI.MAX Trial." *Intl J Cancer* 116:2 (2005): 182–186.

48. Mooney, L.A., A.M. Madsen, D. Tang, et al. "Antioxidant Vitamin Supplementation Reduces Benzo(a)pyrene-DNA Adducts and Potential Cancer Risk in Female Smokers." *Cancer Epidemiol Biomarkers Prev* 14:1 (2005): 237–242. Wright, M.E., S.T. Mayne, R.Z. Stolzenberg-Solomon, et al. "Development of a Comprehensive Dietary Antioxidant Index and Application to Lung Cancer Risk in a Cohort of Male Smokers." *Am J Epidemiol* 160:1 (2004): 68–76.

49. Cameron, E., and L. Pauling. "Supplemental Ascorbate in the Supportive

Treatment of Cancer: Prolongation of Survival Times in Terminal Human Cancer." *Proc Natl Acad Sci U S A* 73 (1976): 3685–3689. Creagan, E.T., C.G. Moertel, J.R. O'Fallon, et al. "Failure of High-dose Vitamin C Therapy to Benefit Patients with Advanced Cancer. A Controlled Trial." *N Engl J Med* 301 (1979): 687–690.

50. Agus, D.B., J.C. Vera, D.W. Golde. "Stromal Cell Oxidation: A Mechanism by which Tumors Obtain Vitamin C." *Cancer Res* 59 (1999): 4555–4558.

51. Chen, Q., M.G. Espey, A.Y. Sun, et al. "Ascorbate in Pharmacologic Concentrations Selectively Generates Ascorbate Radical and Hydrogen Peroxide in Extracellular Fluid in vivo." *Proc Natl Acad Sci U S A* 104:21 (2007): 8749–8754.

52. Chen, Q., M.G. Espey, M.C. Krishna, et al. "Pharmacologic Ascorbic Acid Concentrations Selectively Kill Cancer Cells: Action as a Pro-drug to Deliver Hydrogen Peroxide to Tissues." *Proc Natl Acad Sci U S A* 102:38 (2005): 13604–13609. Casciari, J.J., N.H. Riordan, T.L. Schmidt, et al. "Cytotoxicity of Ascorbate, Lipoic Acid, and Other Antioxidants in Hollow Fibre in vitro Tumours." *Br J Cancer* 84:11 (June 2001): 1544–1550.

53. Komarova, S.V., F.I. Ataullakhanov, R.K. Globus. "Bioenergetics and Mitochondria Transmembrane Potential During Differentiation of Osteoblast." *Am J Physiol Cell Physiol* 279 (2000): C1220–C1229.

54. Cathcart, R.F. "A Unique Function for Ascorbate." *Med Hypotheses* 35 (1991): 32–37. Morre, D.J., F.L. Crare, I.L. Sun, et al. "The Role of Ascorbate in Biomembrane Energetics." *Ann NY Acad Sci* 498 (1987): 153–171.

55. Simone 2nd, C.B., N.L. Simone, V. Simone, et al. "Antioxidants and Other Nutrients Do Not Interfere with Chemotherapy or Radiation Therapy and Can Increase Kill and Increase Survival, Part 1." *Altern Ther Health Med* 13:1 (2007): 22–28. Simone 2nd, C.B., N.L. Simone, V. Simone, et al. "Antioxidants and Other Nutrients Do Not Interfere with Chemotherapy or Radiation Therapy and Can Increase Kill and Increase Survival, Part 2." *Altern Ther Health Med* 13:2 (2007): 40–47.

56. Curhan, G.C., W.C. Willett, E.B. Rimm, et al. "A Prospective Study of the Intake of Vitamins C and B_6, and the Risk of Kidney Stones in Men." *J Urol* 155:6 (1996): 1847–1851.

57. Curhan, G.C., W.C. Willett, F.E. Speizer, et al. "Megadose Vitamin C Consumption Does Not Cause Kidney Stones. Intake of Vitamins B_6 and C and the Risk of Kidney Stones in Women." *J Am Soc Nephrol* 10:4 (April 1999): 840–845.

Chapter 5: Energy Factors for Cancer Patients

1. Warburg, O. "On the Origin of Cancer Cells." *Science* 123:3191 (1956): 309–314.

2. Kagan, V.E., and Y.Y. Tyurina. "Recycling and Redox Cycling of Phenolic Antioxidants." *Ann NY Acad Sci* 854 (November 1998): 425–434. Njus, D., P.M. Kelley, G.J. Harnadek, et al. "Mechanism of Ascorbic Acid Regeneration Mediated by Cytochrome b561." *Ann NY Acad Sci* 493 (1987): 108–119. Chaudiere, J., and R. Ferrari-Iliou. "Intracellular Antioxidants: From Chemical to Biochemical Mechanisms." *Food Chem Toxicol* 37:9–10 (September-October 1999): 949–962.

3. Whiteman, M., H. Tritschler, B. Halliwell. "Protection against Peroxynitrite-dependent Tyrosine Nitration and Alpha 1-antiproteinase Inactivation by Oxidized and Reduced Lipoic Acid." *FEBS Lett* 379 (January 1996): 74–76.

4. Packer, L., K. Kraemer, G. Rimbach G. "Molecular Aspects of Lipoic Acid in the Prevention of Diabetes Complications." *Nutrition* 17 (2001): 888–895. Wollin, S.D., and P.J. Jones. "Alpha-lipoic Acid and Cardiovascular Disease." *J Nutr* 133 (2003): 3327–3330. Duenschede, F., K. Erbes, A. Kircher, et al. "Protection from Hepatic Ischemia/Reperfusion Injury and Improvement of Liver Regeneration by Alpha-lipoic Acid." *Shock* 27 (2007): 644–651. Bilska, A., and L. Wlodek. "Lipoic Acid-The Drug of the Future?" *Pharmacol Rep* 57:5 (2005): 570–577. Lee, E.Y., C.K. Lee, K.U. Lee, et al. "Alpha-lipoic Acid Suppresses the Development of Collagen-induced Arthritis and Protects against Bone Destruction in Mice." *Rheumatol Intl* 27 (2007): 225–233. Manda, K., M. Ueno, T. Moritake, et al. "Radiation-induced Cognitive Dysfunction and Cerebellar Oxidative Stress in Mice: Protective Effect of Alpha-lipoic Acid." *Behav Brain Res* 177 (2007): 7–14. Smith, A.R., S.V. Shenvi, M. Widlansky, et al. "Lipoic Acid as a Potential Therapy for Chronic Diseases Associated with Oxidative Stress." *Curr Med Chem* 11 (2004): 1135–1146.

5. Karpov, L.M., E.D. Dvuzhil'naia, V.I. Savvov, et al. ["S35 Lipoic Acid Distribution and Its Effect on Pyruvate Dehydrogenase Activity in Rats with Walker Carcinoma."] *Vopr Onkol* 23:10 (1977): 87–90.

6. Selvakumar, E., and T.C. Hsieh. "Regulation of Cell Cycle Transition and Induction of Apoptosis in HL-60 Leukemia Cells by Lipoic Acid: Role in Cancer Prevention and Therapy." *J Hematol Oncol* 1 (2008): 4.

7. Pack, R.A., K. Hardy, M.C. Madigan, et al. "Differential Effects of the Antioxidant Alpha-lipoic Acid on the Proliferation of Mitogen-stimulated Peripheral Blood Lymphocytes and Leukaemic T Cells." *Mol Immunol* 38:10 (2002): 733–745.

8. Sokoloski, J.A., W.F. Hodnick, S.T. Mayne, et al. "Induction of the Differentiation of HL-60 Promyelocytic Leukemia Cells by Vitamin E and Other Antioxidants in Combination with Low Levels of Vitamin D3: Possible Relationship to NF-kappaB." *Leukemia* 11:9 (September 1997): 1546–1553. Zhang, W.J., and B. Frei. "Alpha-lipoic Acid Inhibits TNF-alpha-induced NF-kappaB

Activation and Adhesion Molecule Expression in Human Aortic Endothelial Cells." *FASEB J* 15:13 (2001): 2423–2432.

9. Packer, Lester. *The Antioxidant Miracle*. New York: Wiley, 1999.

10. Ho, Y.S., C.S. Lai, H.I. Liu, et al. "Dihydrolipoic Acid Inhibits Skin Tumor Promotion through Anti-inflammation and Anti-oxidation." *Biochem Pharmacol* 73:11 (2007): 1786–1795.

11. Pack, R.A., K. Hardy, M.C. Madigan, et al. "Differential Effects of the Antioxidant Alpha-lipoic Acid on the Proliferation of Mitogen-stimulated Peripheral Blood Lymphocytes and Leukaemic T Cells." *Mol Immunol* 38:10 (2002): 733–745. Wenzel, U., A. Nickel, H. Daniel. "Alpha-lipoic Acid Induces Apoptosis in Human Colon Cancer Cells by Increasing Mitochondrial Respiration with a Concomitant O_2-*-Generation." *Apoptosis* 10 (2005): 359–368. Vig-Varga, E., E.A. Benson, T.L. Limbil, et al. "Alpha-lipoic Acid Modulates Ovarian Surface Epithelial Cell Growth." *Gynecol Oncol* 103 (2006): 45–52.

12. van de Mark, K., J.S. Chen, K. Steliou, et al. "Alpha-lipoic Acid Induces p27Kip-dependent Cell Cycle Arrest in Non-transformed Cell Lines and Apoptosis in Tumor Cell Lines." *J Cell Physiol* 194:3 (March 2003): 325–340.

13. Moungjaroen, J., U. Nimmannit, P.S. Callery, et al. "Reactive Oxygen Species Mediate Caspase Activation and Apoptosis Induced by Lipoic Acid in Human Lung Epithelial Cancer Cells through *Bcl-2* Down-regulation." *J Pharmacol Exp Ther* 319 (2006): 1062–1069.

14. Casciari, J.J., et al. "Cytotoxicity of Ascorbate, Lipoic Acid, and Other Antioxidants in Hollow Fiber in vitro Tumors." *Br J Cancer* 84 (2001): 1544–1550.

15. Wenzel, U., A. Nickel, H. Daniel. "Alpha-lipoic Acid Induces Apoptosis in Human Colon Cancer Cells by Increasing Mitochondrial Respiration with a Concomitant O_2-*-Generation." *Apoptosis* 10 (2005): 359–368.

16. Berger, M., M. Habs, D. Schmahl. ["Effect of Thioctic Acid (Alpha-lipoic Acid) on the Chemotherapeutic Efficacy of Cyclophosphamide and Vincristine Sulfate."] *Arzneimittelforschung* 33:9 (1983): 1286–1288.

17. Dovinova, I., L. Novotny, P. Rauko, et al. "Combined Effect of Lipoic Acid and Doxorubicin in Murine Leukemia." *Neoplasma* 46:4 (1999): 237–241.

18. Ryback, L.P., K. Husain, C. Whitworth, et al. "Dose-dependent Protection by Lipoic Acid against Cisplatin-induced Ototoxicity in Rats: Antioxidant Defense System." *Toxicol Sci* 47:2 (1999): 195–202.

19. Somani, S.M., K. Husain, C. Whitworth, et al. "Dose-dependent Protection by Lipoic Acid against Cisplatin-induced Nephrotoxicity in Rats: Antioxidant Defense System." *Pharmacol Toxicol* 86:5 (2000): 234–241.

20. Balachandar, A.V., K.P. Malarkodi, P. Varalakshmi. "Protective Role of DL

Alpha-lipoic Acid against Adriamycin-induced Cardiac Lipid Peroxidation." *Hum Exp Toxicol* 22 (2003): 249–254. Al-Majed, A.A., A.M. Gdo, O.A. Al-Shabanah, et al. "Alpha-lipoic Acid Ameliorates Myocardial Toxicity Induced by Doxorubicin." *Pharmacol Res* 46 (2002): 499–503.

21. Prahalathan, C., E. Selvakumar, P. Varalakshmi. "Remedial Effect of DL-Alpha-lipoic Acid against Adriamycin-induced Testicular Lipid Peroxidation." *Mol Cell Biochem* 267:1–2 (2004): 209–214.

22. Gedlicka, C., W. Scheithauer, B. Schüll, et al. "Effective Treatment of Oxaliplatin-Induced Cumulative Polyneuropathy with Alpha-Lipoic Acid." *J Clin Oncol* 20 (2002): 3359–3361.

23. Ziegler, D., M. Hanefeld, K.J. Ruhnau, et al. "Treatment of Symptomatic Diabetic Polyneuropathy with the Antioxidant Alpha-lipoic Acid: A 7-Month Multicenter Randomized Controlled Trial. ALADIN III Study Group. ALADIN III Study." *Diabetes Care* 22 (1999): 1296–1301.

24. Jacob, S., E.J. Henriksen, H.J. Tritschler, et al. "Improvement of Insulin-stimulated Glucose-disposal in Type 2 Diabetes after Repeated Parenteral Administration of Thioctic Acid." *Exp Clin Endocrinol Diabetes* 104 (1996): 284–288.

25. Cremer, D.R., R. Rabeler, A. Roberts, et al. "Long-term Safety of Alpha-lipoic Acid (ALA) Consumption: A 2-year Study." *Regul Toxicol Pharmacol* 46 (2006): 193–201.

26. Kamenova, P. "Improvement of Insulin Sensitivity in Patients with Type 2 Diabetes Mellitus after Oral Administration of Alpha-lipoic Acid." *Hormones (Athens)* 5:4 (2006): 251–258.

27. Casciari, J.J., et al. "Cytotoxicity of Ascorbate, Lipoic Acid, and Other Antioxidants in Hollow Fiber in vitro Tumors." *Br J Cancer* 84 (2001): 1544–1550.

28. Sarter, B. "Coenzyme Q_{10} and Cardiovascular Disease: A Review." *J Cardiovasc Nurs* 16:4 (2002): 9–20. Pepe, S., S.F. Marasco, S.J. Haas, et al. "Coenzyme Q_{10} in Cardiovascular Disease." *Mitochondrion* 7:Suppl (2007): S154–S167.

29. Langsjoen, P.H., J.O. Langsjoen, A.M. Langsjoen, et al. "Treatment of Statin Adverse Effects with Supplemental Coenzyme Q_{10} and Statin Drug Discontinuation." *Biofactors* 25 (2005): 147–152.

30. Tomasetti, M., R. Alleva, B. Borghi, et al. "In vivo Supplementation with Coenzyme Q_{10} Enhances the Recovery of Human Lymphocytes from Oxidative DNA Damage." *FASEB J* 15:8 (2001): 1425–1427.

31. Lockwood, K., S. Moesgaard, et al. "Progress on Therapy of Breast Cancer with Vitamin Q_{10} and the Regression of Metastases." *Biochem Biophys Res Commun* 212 (1995): 172–177.

32. Palan, P.R., M.S. Mikhail, D.W. Shaban, et al. "Plasma Concentrations of Coenzyme Q_{10} and Tocopherols in Cervical Intraepithelial Neoplasia and Cervical Cancer." *Eur J Cancer Prev* 12 (2003): 321–326.

33. Mikhail, M.S., et al. "Coenzyme Q_{10} and Alpha-Tocopherol Concentrations in Cervical Intraepithelial Neoplasia and Cervix Cancer." *Obstet Gynecol* 97 (2001): (Abstract)3S.

34. Folkers, K., A. Osterborg, et al. "Activities of Vitamin Q_{10} in Animal Models and a Serious Deficiency in Patients with Cancer." *Biochem Biophys Res Commun* 234 (1997): 296–299.

35. Portakal, O., O. Ozkaya, M. Erden Inal, et al. "Coenzyme Q_{10} Concentrations and Antioxidant Status in Tissues of Breast Cancer Patients." *Clin Biochem* 33 (2000): 279–284.

36. Lockwood, K., S. Moesgaard, T. Hanioka, et al. "Apparent Partial Remission of Breast Cancer in 'High Risk' Patients Supplemented with Nutritional Antioxidants, Essential Fatty Acids and Coenzyme Q_{10}." *Mol Aspects Med* 15:Suppl (1994): S231–S240.

37. Lockwood, K., S. Moesgaard, T. Yamamoto, et al. "Progress on Therapy of Breast Cancer with Vitamin Q_{10} and the Regression of Metastases." *Biochem Biophys Res Commun* 212:1 (1995): 172–177.

38. Rusciani, L., I. Proietti, A. Rusciani, et al. "Low Plasma Coenzyme Q_{10} Levels as an Independent Prognostic Factor for Melanoma Progression." *J Am Acad Dermatol* 54:2 (2006): 234–241. Lockwood, K., S. Moesgaard, et al. "Apparent Partial Remission of Breast Cancer in 'High Risk' Patients Supplemented with Nutritional Antioxidants, Essential Fatty Acids and Coenzyme Q_{10}." *Mol Aspects Med* 15 (1994): S231–S240. Chipperfield, B., and J.R. Chipperfield. "Ubiquinone and Nucleic Acid Concentration in the Heart Muscle of Cancer Patients and Normal Controls." *Clin Chem Acta* 31 (1971): 459–465. Ohhara, H., H. Kanaide, et al. "A Protective Effect of Coenzyme Q_{10} on Ischemia and Reperfusion of the Isolated Perfused Rat Heart." *J Mol Cell Cardiol* 13 (1981): 65–74.

39. Tomasetti, M., R. Alleva, B. Borghi, et al. "In vivo Supplementation with Coenzyme Q_{10} Enhances the Recovery of Human Lymphocytes from Oxidative DNA Damage." *FASEB J* 15:8 (2001): 1425–1427.

40. Nicolson, G.L., and K.A. Conklin. "Reversing Mitochondrial Dysfunction, Fatigue and the Adverse Effects of Chemotherapy of Metastatic Disease by Molecular Replacement Therapy." *Clin Exp Metastasis* 25:2 (2008): 161–169.

41. Judy, W., J. Hall, W. Dugan, et al. "Coenzyme Q_{10} Reduction of Adriamycin Cardiotoxicity." *Biomed Clin Aspects Coenzyme Q* 4 (1984): 231–241.

42. Premkumar, V.G., S. Yuvaraj, K. Vijayasarathy, et al. "Effect of Coenzyme

Q_{10}, Riboflavin and Niacin on Serum CEA and CA 15-3 Levels in Breast Cancer Patients Undergoing Tamoxifen Therapy." *Biol Pharm Bull* 30 (2007): 367–370.

43. Hodges, S., N. Hertz, K. Lockwood, et al. "CoQ_{10}: Could It Have a Role in Cancer Management?" *Biofactors* 9 (1999): 365–370.

44. Ferrante, K.L., J. Shefner, et al. "Tolerance of High-dose (3,000 mg/Day) Coenzyme Q_{10} in ALS." *Neurology* 65:11 (December 2005): 1834–1836.

45. Mizuno, K., M. Tanaka, S. Nozaki, et al. "Antifatigue Effects of Coenzyme Q_{10} During Physical Fatigue." *Nutrition* 24:4 (2008): 293–299.

46. Nuku, K., Y. Matsuoka, T. Yamagishi, et al. "Safety Assessment of PureSorb-Q40 in Healthy Subjects and Serum Coenzyme Q_{10} Level in Excessive Dosing." *J Nutr Sci Vitaminol* 53 (2007): 198–206.

47. Sarter, B. "Coenzyme Q_{10} and Cardiovascular Disease: A Review." *J Cardiovasc Nurs* 16:4 (2002): 9–20. Langsjoen, P.H., J.O. Langsjoen, A.M. Langsjoen, et al. "Treatment of Statin Adverse Effects with Supplemental Coenzyme Q_{10} and Statin Drug Discontinuation." *Biofactors* 25 (2005): 147–152.

48. Pepe, S., S.F. Marasco, S.J. Haas, et al. "Coenzyme Q_{10} in Cardiovascular Disease." *Mitochondrion* 7:Suppl (2007): S154–S167.

49. Premkumar, V.G., S. Yuvaraj, K. Vijayasarathy, et al. "Effect of Coenzyme Q_{10}, Riboflavin and Niacin on Serum CEA and CA 15-3 Levels in Breast Cancer Patients Undergoing Tamoxifen Therapy." *Biol Pharm Bull* 30 (2007): 367–370. Lockwood, K., S. Moesgaard, T. Yamamoto, et al. "Progress on Therapy of Breast Cancer with Vitamin Q_{10} and the Regression of Metastases." *Biochem Biophys Res Commun* 212:1 (1995): 172–177. Lockwood, K., S. Moesgaard, et al. "Apparent Partial Remission of Breast Cancer in 'High Risk' Patients Supplemented with Nutritional Antioxidants, Essential Fatty Acids and Coenzyme Q_{10}." *Mol Aspects Med* 15 (1994): S231–S240.

50. Hagen, T.M., R. Moreau, J.H. Suh, et al. "Mitochondrial Decay in the Aging Rat Heart: Evidence for Improvement by Dietary Supplementation with Acetyl-L-carnitine and/or Lipoic Acid." *Ann NY Acad Sci* 959 (April 2002): 491–507. Hagen, T.M., J. Liu, J. Lykkesfeldt, et al. "Feeding Acetyl-L-carnitine and Lipoic Acid to Old Rats Significantly Improves Metabolic Function while Decreasing Oxidative Stress." *Proc Natl Acad Sci U S A* 99 (2002): 1870–1875. Shen, W., J. Hao, C. Tian, et al. "A Combination of Nutriments Improves Mitochondrial Biogenesis and Function in Skeletal Muscle of Type 2 Diabetic Goto-Kakizaki Rats." *PLoS ONE* 3 (2008): e2328.

51. Singh, R.B., M.A. Niaz, P. Agarwal, et al. "A Randomised, Double-blind, Placebo-controlled Trial of L-Carnitine in Suspected Acute Myocardial Infarction." *Postgrad Med J* 72 (1996): 45–50. Ferrari, R., E. Merli, G. Cicchitelli, et

al. "Therapeutic Effects of L-Carnitine and Propionyl-L-carnitine on Cardiovascular Diseases: A Review." *Ann NY Acad Sci* 1033 (2004): 79–91. The Investigators of the Study on Propionyl-L-Carnitine in Chronic Heart Failure. "Study on Propionyl-L-carnitine in Chronic Heart Failure." *Eur Heart J* 20 (1999): 70–76. Cherchi, A., C. Lai, F. Angelino, et al. "Effects of L-Carnitine on Exercise Tolerance in Chronic Stable Angina: A Multicenter, Double-blind, Randomized, Placebo-controlled Crossover Study." *Intl J Clin Pharmacol Ther Toxicol* 23 (1985): 569–572. Poorabbas, A., F. Fallah, J. Bagdadchi, et al. "Determination of Free L-Carnitine Levels in Type II Diabetic Women With and Without Complications." *Eur J Clin Nutr* 61 (2007): 892–895.

52. Fan, J.P., H.S. Kim, G.D. Han. "Induction of Apoptosis by L:-carnitine through Regulation of Two Main Pathways in Hepa1c1c 7 Cells." *Amino Acids* (April 2008).

53. Cruciani, R.A., E. Dvorkin, P. Homel, et al. "Safety, Tolerability and Symptom Outcomes Associated with L-Carnitine Supplementation in Patients with Cancer, Fatigue, and Carnitine Deficiency: A Phase I/II Study." *J Pain Symptom Manage* 32 (2006): 551–559. De Grandis, D. "Acetyl-L-carnitine for the Treatment of Chemotherapy-induced Peripheral Neuropathy: A Short Review." *CNS Drugs* 21 (2007): 39–43. "The L-Carnitine Ecocardiografia Digitalizzata Infarto Miocardico (CEDIM) Trial." *J Am Coll Cardiol* 26:2 (1995): 380–387. Pisano, C., G. Pratesi, D. Laccabue, et al. "Paclitaxel and Cisplatin-induced Neurotoxicity: A Protective Role of Acetyl-L-Carnitine." *Clin Cancer Res* 9 (2003): 5756–5767.

54. Hathcock, J.N., and A. Shao. "Risk Assessment for Carnitine." *Regul Toxicol Pharmacol* 46:1 (2006): 23–28.

Chapter 6: More Rejuvenating Factors for Cancer Patients

1. de Escobar, G.M., MJ. Obregon, F.E. del Rey. "Iodine Deficiency and Brain Development in the First Half of Pregnancy." *Public Health Nutr* 10:12A (2007): 1554–1570.

2. Patrick, L. "Iodine: Deficiency and Therapeutic Considerations." *Altern Med Rev* 13:2 (2008): 116–127.

3. Goehring, C., and A. Morabia. "Epidemiology of Benign Breast Disease, with Special Attention to Histologic Types." *Epidemiol Rev* 19 (1997): 310–327.

4. Hartmann, L.C., T.A. Sellers, M.H. Frost, et al. "Benign Breast Disease and the Risk of Breast Cancer." *N Engl J Med* 353 (2005): 229–237.

5. Baer, H.J., S.J. Schnitt, J.L. Connolly. "Adolescent Diet and Incidence of Proliferative Benign Breast Disease." *Cancer Epidemiol Biomarkers Prev* 12:11 Part 1 (November 2003): 1159–1167.

6. Eskin, B.A., D.G. Bartuska, M. Dunn, et al. "Mammary Gland Dysplasia in Iodine Deficiency." *JAMA* 200 (1967): 115–119. Eskin, B.A. "Iodine Metabolism and Cancer." *Trans NY Acad Sci* 32 (1970): 911–947. Eskin, B.A. "Iodine and Mammary Cancer." *Adv Exp Med Biol* 91 (1977): 293–304.

7. Ghent, W.R., B.A. Eskin, D.A. Low, et al. "Iodine Replacement in Fibrocystic Disease of the Breast." *Can J Surg* 36:5 (1993): 453–460.

8. Patrick, L. "Iodine: Deficiency and Therapeutic Considerations." *Altern Med Rev* 13:2 (2008): 116–127.

9. Stoddard 2nd, F.R., A.D. Brooks, B.A. Eskin, et al. "Iodine Alters Gene Expression in the MCF7 Breast Cancer Cell Line: Evidence for an Anti-estrogen Effect of Iodine." *Intl J Med Sci* 5:4 (July 2008): 189–196.

10. Kogai, T., K. Taki, G.A. Brent. "Enhancement of Sodium/Iodide Symporter Expression in Thyroid and Breast Cancer." *Endocr Relat Cancer* 13:3 (2006): 797–826.

11. Shrivastava, A., M. Tiwari, R.A. Sinha, et al. "Molecular Iodine Induces Caspase-independent Apoptosis in Human Breast Carcinoma Cells Involving the Mitochondria-mediated Pathway." *J Biol Chem* 281 (2006): 19762–19771.

12. Smyth, P.A. "Role of Iodine in Antioxidant Defence in Thyroid and Breast Disease." *Biofactors* 19 (2003): 121–130.

13. Anguiano, B., P. Garcia-Solis, G. Delgado, et al. "Uptake and Gene Expression with Antitumoral Doses of Iodine in Thyroid and Mammary Gland: Evidence that Chronic Administration has No Harmful Effects." *Thyroid* 17:9 (2007): 851–859.

14. Giray, B., F. Hincal, T. Tezic, et al. "Status of Selenium and Antioxidant Enzymes of Goitrous Children is Lower Than Healthy Controls and Non-goitrous Children with High Iodine Deficiency." *Biol Trace Elem Res* 82 (2001): 35–52.

15. Zimmermann, M.B., and J. Kohrle. "The Impact of Iron and Selenium Deficiencies on Iodine and Thyroid Metabolism: Biochemistry and Relevance to Public Health." *Thyroid* 12 (2002): 867–878.

16. Ghent, W.R., B.A. Eskin, D.A. Low, et al. "Iodine Replacement in Fibrocystic Disease of the Breast." *Can J Surg* 36:5 (1993): 453–460. Kessler, J.H. "The Effect of Supraphysiologic Levels of Iodine on Patients with Cyclic Mastalgia." *Breast J* 10 (2004): 328–336.

17. Beard, J. "The Action of Trypsin upon the Living Cells of Jensen's Mouse Tumor." *Br Med J* 4 (1906): 140–141.

18. Wiggin, F.H. "Case of Multiple Fibrosarcoma of the Tongue with Remarks on the Use of Trypsin and Amylopsin in the Treatment of Malignant Disease."

JAMA 47 (1906): 2003–2008. Campbell, J.T. "Trypsin Treatment of a Case of Malignant Disease." *JAMA* 48 (1907): 225–226. Cutfield, A. "Trypsin Treatment in Malignant Disease." *Br Med J* 5 (1907): 525. Goeth, R.A. "Pancreatic Treatment of Cancer with Report of a Cure." *JAMA* 48 (1907): 1030. Little, W.L. "A Case of Malignant Tumor with Treatment." *JAMA* 50 (1908): 1724.

19. Beard, J. *The Enzyme Treatment of Cancer.* London: Chatto and Windus, 1911.

20. Kelley, W.D., and F. Rohe. *Cancer: Curing the Incurable without Surgery, Chemotherapy, or Radiation.* Bonita, CA: New Century Promotions, 2005, pp. 3–13. Gonzalez, N.J., and L.L. Isaacs. "Evaluation of Pancreatic Proteolytic Enzyme Treatment of Adenocarcinoma of the Pancreas, with Nutrition and Detoxification Support." *Nutr Cancer* 33:2 (1999): 117–124. Gonzalez, N.J., and L.L. Isaacs. "Enzyme Therapy and Cancer: A Collection of Case Reports." *Altern Ther Health Med* 13:1 (January-February 2007): 46–55.

21. Leipner, J., and R. Saller. "Systemic Enzyme Therapy in Oncology: Effect and Mode of Action." *Drugs* 59:4 (2000): 769–780.

22. Stauder, G.; Enzyme Research Medical Society, Geretsried, Germany. "Pharmacological Effects of Oral Enzyme Combinations." *Cas Lek Cesk* 134:19 (October 1995): 620–624.

23. Desser, L., et al. "Oral Therapy with Proteolytic Enzymes Decreases Excessive TGF-beta Levels in Human Blood." *Cancer Chemother Pharmacol* 47 (2001): S10–S15.

24. Fidlerm, I.J. "Critical Factors in the Biology of Human Cancer Metastasis: Twenty-eighth GHA Clowes Memorial Award Lecture." *Cancer Res* 50:19 (1990): 6130–6138.

25. Dvorak, H.F., D.R. Senger, A.M. Dvorak. "Fibrin as a Component of the Tumor Stroma: Origins and Biological Significance." *Cancer Metastasis Rev* 2:1 (1983): 41–73. Costantini, V., and L.R. Zacharski. "The Role of Fibrin in Tumor Metastasis." *Cancer Metastasis Rev* 11:3 (1992): 283–290.

26. Yamamoto, K., S. Omata, T. Ohnishi, et al. "In vivo Effects of Proteases on Cell Surface Architecture and Cell Proliferation in the Liver." *Cancer Res* 33 (1973): 567–572.

27. Wald, M., et al. "Mixture of Trypsin, Chymotrypsin and Papain Reduces Formation of Metastases and Extended Survival Time of C57Bl6 Mice with Syngeneic Melanoma B16." *Cancer Chemother Pharmacol* 47 (2001): S16–S22.

28. Gonzalez, N.J., and L.L. Isaacs. "Evaluation of Pancreatic Proteolytic Enzyme Treatment of Adenocarcinoma of the Pancreas, with Nutrition and Detoxification Support." *Nutr Cancer* 33:2 (1999): 117–124.

29. National Cancer Institute and Surveillance Epidemiology and End Results (SEER) Program. *Pancreas* (1988–1992): 104–107.

30. Pour, P.M., et al. "Pancreatic Enzyme Extract Improves Survival in Murine Pancreatic Cancer." *Pancreas* 28 (2001): 401–412.

31. Desser, L., et al. "Oral Enzymes as Additive Cancer Therapy." *Intl J Immunother* 17 (2001): 153–161.

32. Beuth, J., et al. "Impact of Complementary Oral Enzyme Application on the Postoperative Treatment Results of Breast Cancer Patients—Results of an Epidemiological Multicentre Retrolective Cohort Study." *Cancer Chemother Pharmacol* 47 (2001): S45–S54.

33. Popiela, T., J. Kulig, H. Jurgen, et al. "Influence of a Complementary Treatment with Oral Enzymes on Patients with Colorectal Cancers—An Epidemiological Retroactive Cohort Study." *Cancer Chemother Pharmacol* 47 (2001): S55–S63.

34. Yamamoto, H., et al. "Association of Trypsin Expression with Tumour Progression and Matrilysin Expression in Human Colorectal Cancer." *J Pathol* 199 (2003): 176–184.

35. Baak, J.P.A., H. Korner, E.A. Janssen, et al. "Trypsin in Colorectal Cancer: Molecular Biological Mechanisms of Proliferation, Invasion, and Metastasis." *J Pathol* 209 (2006): 147–156. Saruc, M., S. Standop, J. Standop, et al. "Pancreatic Enzyme Extract Improves Survival in Murine Pancreatic Cancer." *Pancreas* 28:4 (2004): 401–412.

36. Seo, T., W.M. Blaner, R.J. Deckelbaum. "Omega-3 Fatty Acids Molecular Approaches to Optimal Biological Outcomes." *Current Opin Lipidol* 16 (2005): 11–18.

37. Larsson, S.C., M. Kumlin, M. Ingelman-Sundberg, et al. "Dietary Long-chain n-3 Fatty Acids for the Prevention of Cancer: A Review of Potential Mechanisms." *Am J Clin Nutr* 79 (2004): 935–945. Roynette, C.E., P.C. Calder, Y.M. Dupertuis, et al. "n-3 Polyunsaturated Fatty Acids and Colon Cancer Prevention." *Clin Nutr* 23 (2004): 139–151.

38. Terry, P.D., T.E. Rohan, A. Wolk. "Intakes of Fish and Marine Fatty Acids and the Risks of Cancers of the Breast and Prostate and of Other Hormone-related Cancers: A Review of the Epidemiologic Evidence." *Am J Clin Nutr* 77 (2003): 532–543.

39. Ferguson, L.R., and M. Phipott. "Immunonutrition and Cancer." *Mutat Res* 551:1–2 (2004): 29–42. Calder, P.C. "Dietary Modification of Inflammation with Lipids." *Proc Nutr Soc* 61 (2002): 345–358. Calder, P.C., and R.F. Grimble. "Polyunsaturated Fatty Acids, Inflammation and Immunity." *Eur J Clin Nutr* 56:Suppl (2002): S14–S19. Koch, T., et al. "Omega-3 Fatty Acids Improve Liver and Pancreas Function in Postoperative Cancer Patients." *Intl J Cancer* 111 (2004): 611–616.

40. Hardman, W.E. "Omega-3 Fatty Acids to Augment Cancer Therapy." *J Nutr* 132 (2002): 3508S–3512S.

41. Koch, T., et al. "Omega-3 Fatty Acids Improve Liver and Pancreas Function in Postoperative Cancer Patients." *Intl J Cancer* 111 (2004): 611–616.

42. Shahidi, F., and H. Miralialbari. "Omega-3 (n-3) Fatty Acids in Health and Disease: Part 1—Cardiovascular Disease and Cancer." *J Med Food* 7:4 (2004): 387–401.

43. Rose, D.P., and J.M. Connolly. "Omega-3 Fatty Acids as Cancer Chemopreventative Agents." *J Natl Cancer Inst* 83 (1999): 217–244.

44. Gonzalez, M.J. "Fish Oil, Lipid Peroxidation and Mammary Tumor Growth." *J Am Coll Nutr* 14:4 (August 1995): 325–335.

45. Autier, P., and S. Gandini. "Vitamin D Supplementation and Total Mortality: A Meta-analysis of Randomized Controlled Trials." *Arch Intern Med* 167:16 (September 2007): 1730–1737.

46. Lappe, J.M., D. Travers-Gustafson, K.M. Davies, et al. "Vitamin D and Calcium Supplementation Reduces Cancer Risk: Results of a Randomized Trial." *Am J Clin Nutr* 85 (2007): 1586–1591.

47. Autier, P., and S. Gandini. "Vitamin D Supplementation and Total Mortality: A Meta-analysis of Randomized Controlled Trials." *Arch Intern Med* 167:16 (2007): 1730–1737.

48. Grau, M.V., J.A. Baron, R.S. Sandler, et al. "Vitamin D, Calcium Supplementation, and Colorectal Adenomas: Results of a Randomized Trial." *J Natl Cancer Inst* 95:23 (December 2003): 1765–1771.

49. Gorham, E.D., C.F. Garland, F.C. Garland, et al. "Optimal Vitamin D Status for Colorectal Cancer Prevention: A Quantitative Meta-analysis." *Am J Prev Med* 32:3 (March 2007): 210–216.

50. Bischoff-Ferrari, H.A., E. Giovannucci, W.C. Willett, et al. "Estimation of Optimal Serum Concentrations of 25-Hydroxyvitamin D for Multiple Health Outcomes." *Am J Clin Nutr* 84:1 (2006): 18–28.

51. de Moreno de LeBlanc, A., C Matar, G. Perdigon. "The Application of Probiotics in Cancer." *Br J Nutr* 98:Suppl 1 (October 2007): S105–S110.

52. Rescigno, M. "The Pathogenic Role of Intestinal Flora in IBD and Colon Cancer." *Curr Drug Targets* 9:5 (May 2008): 395–403.

53. Rao, C.V., M.E. Sanders, C. Indranie, et al. "Prevention of Colonic Preneoplastic Lesions by the Probiotic *Lactobacillus acidophilus* NCFMTM in F344 Rats." *Intl J Oncol* 14:5 (1999): 939–944.

54. El-Nezami, H.S., N.N. Polychronaki, J. Ma, et al. "Probiotic Supplementa-

tion Reduces a Biomarker for Increased Risk of Liver Cancer in Young Men from Southern China." *Am J Clin Nutr* 83:5 (May 2006): 1199–1203.

55. Osterlund, P., T. Ruotsalainen, R. Korpela, et al. "*Lactobacillus* Supplementation for Diarrhoea Related to Chemotherapy of Colorectal Cancer: A Randomised Study." *Br J Cancer* 97:8 (October 2007): 1028–1034.

56. Rafter, J. "Probiotics and Colon Cancer." *Best Pract Res Clin Gastroenterol* 17:5 (2003): 849–859.

57. Matzno, S., Y. Yamaguchi, T. Akiyoshi, et al. "An Attempt to Evaluate the Effect of Vitamin K$_3$ Using as an Enhancer of Anti-cancer Agents." *Biol Pharm Bull* 31:6 (2008): 1270–1273.

58. Otsuka, M., N. Kato, R.X. Shao, et al. "Vitamin K$_2$ Inhibits the Growth and Invasiveness of Hepatocellular Carcinoma Cells via Protein Kinase A Activation." *Hepatology* 40:1 (July 2004): 243–251.

59. Hitomi, M., F. Yokoyama, Y. Kita, et al. "Antitumor Effects of Vitamins K$_1$, K$_2$ and K$_3$ on Hepatocellular Carcinoma in vitro and in vivo." *Intl J Oncol* 26:3 (2005): 713–720. Mizuta, T., I. Ozaki, Y. Eguchi, et al. "The Effect of Menatetrenone, a Vitamin K$_2$ Analog, on Disease Recurrence and Survival in Patients with Hepatocellular Carcinoma after Curative Treatment: A Pilot Study." *Cancer* 106:4 (February 2006): 867–872.

60. Shibayama-Imazu, T., T. Aiuchi, K. Nakaya. "Vitamin K$_2$-mediated Apoptosis in Cancer Cells: Role of Mitochondrial Transmembrane Potential." *Vitam Horm* 78 (2008): 211–226. Shibayama-Imazu, T., S. Sakairi, A. Watanabe, et al. "Vitamin K($_2$) Selectively Induced Apoptosis in Ovarian TYK-nu and Pancreatic MIA PaCa-2 Cells Out of Eight Solid Tumor Cell Lines Through a Mechanism Different from Geranylgeraniol." *J Cancer Res Clin Oncol* 129:1 (January 2003): 1–11. Sakagami, H., K. Satoh, Y. Hakeda, et al. "Apoptosis-inducing Activity of Vitamin C and Vitamin K." *Cell Mol Biol* (*Noisy-le-grand*) 46:1 (February 2000): 129–143. Ogawa, M., S. Nakai, A. Deguchi, et al. "Vitamins K$_2$, K$_3$ and K$_5$ Exert Antitumor Effects on Established Colorectal Cancer in Mice by Inducing Apoptotic Death of Tumor Cells." *Intl J Oncol* 31:2 (August 2007): 323–331.

Index

About the Authors

Michael J. González, DSc, Ph.D., is professor at the Nutrition Program, School of Public Health, Medical Sciences Campus, University of Puerto Rico. He earned a Bachelor's degree in Biology and Chemistry (Catholic University) and Master's degrees in Cellular Biology and Biophysics (Nova University) and in Nutrition and Public Health (University of Puerto Rico). He also has doctorates in Health Sciences (Lafayette University) and in Nutritional Biochemistry and Cancer Biology (Michigan State University). He completed a post-doctoral fellowship in Geriatrics at the School of Medicine, University of Puerto Rico. Dr. González is a Fellow of the American College of Nutrition and has authored over 100 scientific publications. He has several research awards for his work on nutrition and cancer. As a consultant for several companies, he has been responsible for designing formulations of nutritional supplements and pharmaceutical products. At present, he is a consultant for the Center for the Improvement of Human Functioning, in Wichita, Kansas. He is currently co-director of the RECNAC II project, and research director of the InBioMed Project Initiative.

Jorge R. Miranda-Massari, PharmD, is professor at the School of Pharmacy, Medical Sciences Campus, University of Puerto Rico, and a registered pharmacist. He earned two Bachelor's degrees at the University of Puerto Rico, in Science and in Pharmacy. After earning a doctorate in Pharmacy at the Philadelphia College of Pharmacy and Science, he completed a post-doctoral fellowship in Clinical Pharmacokinetics at the University of North Carolina. He obtained post-doctoral training in Pharmaceutical Care in Nephrology from the

University of Pittsburgh, as well as in Clinical Anti-Coagulation from the Medical College of Virginia. Author of numerous scientific publications, Dr. Miranda-Massari is a consultant for the Center for the Improvement for the Human Functioning, in Wichita, Kansas. He is also director of the education branch of the InBioMed Project and clinical research director of the RECNAC II project, specializing in cancer research. He is the creator of the first course in integrative medicine and the Advanced Practicum in Integrative Medicine at the University of Puerto Rico's School of Pharmacy.

Andrew W. Saul, Ph.D., is assistant editor of the *Journal of Orthomolecular Medicine* and the author of *Fire Your Doctor!* (Basic Health, 2005) and *Doctor Yourself* (Basic Health, 2003). He is co-author (with Steve Hickey, Ph.D.) of *Vitamin C: The Real Story* (Basic Health, 2008) and has also written two books with nutritional medicine pioneer Abram Hoffer, Ph.D.: *The Vitamin Cure for Alcoholism* (Basic Health, 2009) and *Orthomolecular Medicine for Everyone* (Basic Health, 2008). *Psychology Today* named him one of seven natural health pioneers in 2006, and he was featured in the 2008 documentary film *Food Matters* (www.food matters.tv). His educational, non-commercial, peer-reviewed website, DoctorYourself.com, welcomes thousands of visitors each day.

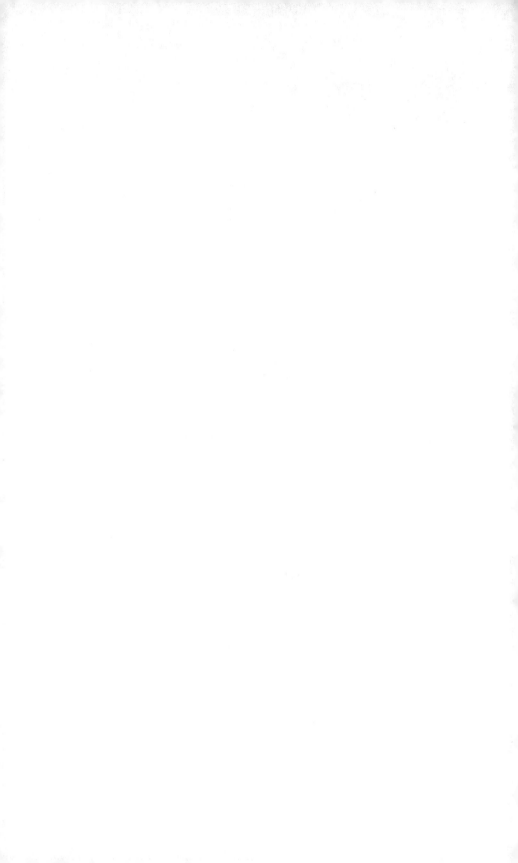

www.ingramcontent.com/pod-product-compliance
Lightning Source LLC
Jackson TN
JSHW011403130125
77033JS00023B/817